GREEN & NATURAL

Skin Care Recipes

Copyright 2011

Pippen

Library of Congress -in-Publication Data
September 2011

The recipes in this book are all made with easily obtained ingredients that are generally accepted to be safe and effective. Individual reactions to the contained ingredients can vary. It is not possible to predict how any individual will react to a particular recipe, treatment, or ingredient. As with any personal care product common sense should be used when creating these recipes. The reader should consult a qualified physician before using any ingredient or created recipe in this book. The enclosed materials are for informational purposes only and the reader accepts all responsibility for determining the effectiveness and usefulness of all included items. Neither the author nor the publisher accepts and liability for the actions of the reader nor for any reactions caused by the use of the contents and ingredients.

GREEN & NATURAL

Skin Care Recipes

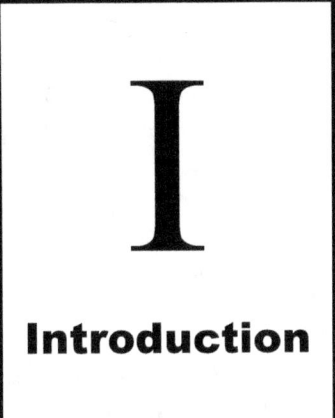

I

Introduction

A walk down the personal care product aisles in your local store can be a lot of fun. There seems to be a product available for just about any need, issue, or desire. Even with such a huge selection, when you start going through each one, you will often find that the exact product you need just is not there.

The products in the personal care aisle are created for everyone, not for the individual. You often know exactly what you want and the results you desire, but because each of us is different with slightly different needs and preferences these products never quite measure up to our expectations.

There is a solution. A cost effective, natural solution customized just for you. Many people do not realize that with key ingredients easily obtained from your grocery store, yard, and kitchen, they can make an entire personal care product line of their own. Better yet, they can make them with fewer unnatural additives. By following simple recipes, a lot like those in a cook book, you can create your very own personal care line. This line will be customized to meet your exact needs. Best yet, this line costs only pennies compared to those items you find in the personal care aisle!

The recipes and alternative ingredient list in this book will help you start creating a personal care line custom suited to your wants, preference, and needs.

You can have the fun and excitement of creating your very own soaps, lotions, make up and cleaners.

➤ You can save hundreds of dollars a year by creating the exact products that you and your family want and need for a fraction of the money you will pay for pre-prepared products.

➤ You can address personal issues, problems, and needs in a way that is focused entirely on you.

➤ You can create a healthier life for your family by using all-natural ingredients.

➤ You can even start your own line of personal care products to share with friends, family, and the world!

Each chapter of the book will provide you with some recipes that are the core products you will use to fill your personal care cabinets. Each of these can be expanded and customized to suit your personal needs. The appendix includes an ingredient list that explains the expected benefit of each ingredient. This list provides you with a basis for customizing each recipe, and beginning to create your own brand new products!

This book is all about experimenting to determine what is best for you! The recipes included are all customizable by exchanging the ingredients I use with the ones you prefer from the ingredient list. I change the recipes continuously to suit the time of year, my personal preferences or even which member of my family is likely to use a particular product. Remember, no two people have exactly the same needs. Each year I try to make a personal care gift pack for each person in my extended family. These gifts are fantastic for holidays and special events since they are created especially for the person receiving the package! These personalized products would cost you hundreds of dollars at a customized shop and still not provide the same benefits as those items you create in your own kitchen.

Now you can have those costly, personalized products that you see in the store but are unwilling to try or that you do buy, much to the detriment of your wallet! You can have these products for just pennies and now, you can provide these same products for you friends and family!

CHAPTER 1

Mineral Makeup

Mineral make up has been used for hundreds, even thousands of years across the globe. Over the last few years, interest in this natural skin colorant has undergone a tremendous boost. Many companies have developed lines of mineral makeup. Each touts the benefits of their line over the next. Whether one is better than another is a matter of opinion and I am not going to express mine here!

What I am going to do is tell you a few of the benefits all of these lines (and home made mineral makeup) offer to you. Then, I will show you the recipe I use to make mineral make up at home for myself, my daughter, my daughter's classmates and friends and even some of my friends and family. I like the make up that I make at home, love that I can feel comfortable having 'girl's day' with my 9 year old and her friends without worrying that I am ruining their skin, and especially love that it costs me pennies to make a years supply of makeup for everyone!

Mineral makeup is a wholly natural make up product created mostly from powdered minerals. The benefits of mineral make up are numerous but the most influential factor to most people is that it is 100% natural.

BENEFITS:

- Mineral makeup is made from zinc and titanium dioxide so it is a natural sunscreen. Depending on how much you use SPF can range from 10 to 20.

- Mineral makeup is typically water resistant. That is not to say water proof but it does last much better while swimming or during water sports than many other make up products.

- Mineral makeup is long-lasting, bearing up better to long days, outdoor activity, and even naps than more traditional make up products.

- Mineral makeup contains ingredients that have special properties of their own. In addition to offering a natural sun screen, you receive the side-benefits of each ingredient. If you look at the recipe for mineral base, you will see that zinc oxide is a main component. Zinc oxide has natural anti-inflammatory properties so the make up you make with zinc oxide will too!

- When applied correctly, the coverage offered by mineral make up is light weight and complete. This makes it perfect for all skin types – from young to old, oily to dry and everything in between.

- Mineral make up is non-comedogenic and (unless you add oils to the recipe) oil free! This means it is less harmful and irritating to your skin. Some makers say it is so clean you can even sleep in it!

- Mineral make up is all natural and the ingredients (unless you add oils to the recipe) do not go bad. That means you do not have to add any preservatives to the mix making it healthier and more natural than the next makeup!

- Mineral make up is fast and easy to apply.

- Mineral make up is VERY inexpensive to make at home.

Base or Foundation

Base or foundation is applied all over the face to create a smooth texture, even skin tone, and flawless finish.

- ➤ 4 tsp   Micronized Titanium Dioxide

- ➤ 1 ½ tsp   Bismuth Oxychloride

- ➤ 2 tsp   Zinc Oxide – Low Micron

- ➤ ½ tsp   Magnesium Stearate

Mix base ingredients by blending well. You can use a mortar / pestle, metal spoon and bowl, or food processor to blend the ingredients.

Slowly add the pigment colorant to the mix.

+/- to preference

- ➤ ¼ tsp   Yellow Iron Oxide

- ➤ Pinch   Brown Iron Oxide

- ➤ Pinch   Red Iron Oxide

- ➤ ½ tsp   Sericite Mica - matte or translucent finish to suit final goals

You can change the tint of the final product to suit your skin tone and color preferences.

For darker shades add more of any of the iron oxides.

For lighter shades add more titanium dioxide or some serecite mica.

Some people have reported that Bismuth Oxychloride causes irritation and redness. If you have sensitive skin or develop a reaction to the recipe, you may try using less or no Bismuth Oxychloride in your recipe.

Some people might want to experiment with different color additives to correct or address certain problems. You could start with:

Yellow Oxide   Brightens dull complexions and counteracts redness.

Chromium Oxide Green   Counters redness from rosacea, acne, or irritated skin.

Ultramarine Violet   Counters yellow or sallow skin tones; minimizes yellowish bruises.

Ultramarine Blue   Counters orange tones that may result from sunless tanning products.

LIQUID APPLICATION – some people prefer a bit more moisture in their makeup or like a liquid application more than a dry application. We make a liquid application by adding the powder mixture to our preferred moisturizer. The consistency of the liquid application is entirely a matter of preference. You will want to experiment by slowly adding the mineral mixture to your favorite moisturizer until you achieve the consistency and coverage amount you desire. The consistency ranges from full coverage matt to a light weight tinted moisturizer.

Mineral Veil – Finish Powder

Mineral Veil is also called a finish powder and gives the face a translucent glow. It is applied on top of all other makeup.

- ➢ 3 tsp   Sericite Mica – Matte
- ➢ 1 tsp   Corn Starch
- ➢ ½ tsp   Boron Nitrate
- ➢ ½ tsp   Magnesium Stearate

Mix base ingredients by blending well. You can use a mortar / pestle, metal spoon and bowl, or food processor to blend the ingredients.

Slowly add the pigment colorant to the mix.

+/- to preference

- ➢ Pinch   Yellow Iron Oxide
- ➢ Pinch   Pink
- ➢ Pinch   Brown Iron Oxide

You can change the tint of the final product to suit your skin tone and color preferences.

For darker shades add more of any of the iron oxides.

For lighter shades add more Corn Starch.

Mineral Make Up – Concealer

A concealer is similar to a foundation in composition with a few simple modifications. Concealer tends to be a couple of shades lighter than your foundation, provides more coverage and is more matte in finish.

- ½ tbsp   Micronized Titanium Dioxide
- ½ tbsp   Serecite Mica – Matte
- ¼ tbsp   Magnesium Stearate

Mix base ingredients by blending well. You can use a mortar / pestle, metal spoon and bowl, or food processor to blend the ingredients.

Slowly add the pigment colorant to the mix.

+/- to preference

- 1/16 tbsp   Yellow Iron Oxide
- Pinch   Light Red or Orange Iron Oxide

You can change the tint of the final product to suit your skin tone and color preferences.

For darker shades add more of any of the iron oxides.

For lighter shades add more titanium dioxide or some serecite mica.

Some people might want to experiment with different color additives to correct or address certain problems. You could start with:

Yellow Oxide   Brightens dull complexions or counteracts redness.

Chromium Oxide Green   Counters redness from rosacea, acne, or irritated skin.

| Ultramarine Violet | Counters yellow or sallow skin tones; minimizes yellowish bruises. |
| Ultramarine Blue | Counters orange tones that may result from sunless tanning products. |

LIQUID APPLICATION

Some people prefer a bit more moisture in their makeup or like a liquid application more than a dry application. We make a liquid application by adding the powder mixture to our preferred moisturizer. The consistency of the liquid application is entirely a matter of preference. You will want to experiment by slowly adding the powder mixture to your favorite moisturizer until you achieve the consistency and coverage amount you desire.

Concealer often needs to be a bit heavier in weight. To create a heavier blend, you may want to try adding more mineral to the moisturizer or use a very heavy moisturizer as the base.

APPLICATION – DRY

To apply concealer in dry or powder form, first apply your foundation then use a small brush to apply the concealer directly to problem areas. Use a larger "Kabuki" brush to blend.

APPLICATION – WET

To apply concealer wet, put a small amount in the palm of your hand, add a small amount of water or moisturizer as desired, and apply with a brush or a sponge to problem areas. By applying wet, you can target larger problem areas. Allow concealer to dry after application. Apply powdered foundation over the concealer to blend and finish.

Bronzer

A bronzer gives extra color where the sun hits the face. The sun leaves a bronze or rosy hue behind. The bronzer gives you the ability to infuse a fresh, healthy glow to your skin without the dangers of spending the day in the sun.

- ➤ 2 tsp   Micronized Titanium Dioxide

- ➤ 1/3 tsp   Magnesium Stearate

Mix base ingredients by blending well. You can use a mortar / pestle, metal spoon and bowl, or food processor to blend the ingredients.

Slowly add the pigment colorant to the mix.

+/- to preference

- ➤ ½ tsp   Yellow Iron Oxide

- ➤ ½ tsp   Brown Iron Oxide

- ➤ ½ tsp   Red Iron Oxide

- ➤ 1 tsp   Sericite Mica – pearl finish

- ➤ ½ tsp   Bronze mica

You can change the tint of the final product to suit your skin tone and color preferences.

For darker shades add more of any of the iron oxides.

For lighter shades add more titanium dioxide or serecite mica.

Mineral Make Up – Eye Shadow

Eye Shadow is used to give extra attention to the eyes.

- ➢ 1 tbsp   Micronized Titanium Dioxide

- ➢ ½ tsp   Magnesium Stearate

- ➢ 1 tsp   Sericite Mica – Pearl or Matte as preferred

  Pearl Sericite will give you a shimmer effect eye shadow

  Matte Sericite will give you a low luster eye shadow

Mix base ingredients by blending well. You can use a mortar / pestle, metal spoon and bowl, or food processor to blend the ingredients.

Slowly add the pigment colorant to the mix.

+/- to preference

- ➢ ½ tsp   Iron Oxide color of your choice.

- Start with ½ tsp and increase until desired color is obtained

- We enjoy mixing multiple colors to attain a shadow that is specific to us. If you custom mix your shadow to your personal preference – DO NOT forget to write down what you did so you can repeat it later.

You can change the tint of the final product to suit your skin tone and color preferences.

For darker shades add more of any of the iron oxides.

For lighter shades add more titanium dioxide or some serecite mica.

Mineral Make Up - Blush

Blush is used to accent the cheekbones and provide a healthy color to the face.

- ➢ 2 ¾ tsp   Sericite Mica
- ➢ 1/4 tsp   Micronized Titanium Dioxide
- ➢ 1/16 tsp   Arrowroot Powder

Mix base ingredients by blending well. You can use a mortar / pestle, metal spoon and bowl, or food processor to blend the ingredients.

Slowly add the pigment colorant to the mix.

+/- to preference

- ➢ 1/16 tsp   Red Iron Oxide

- • Start with 1/16 tsp and increase until desired color is obtained

- • We enjoy mixing multiple colors to attain a shadow that is specific to us. If you custom mix your shadow to your personal preference – DO NOT forget to write down what you did so you can repeat it later.

CHAPTER

2

Facial Soaps & Cleansers

Every inch of your skin is important but perhaps the most important is the facial skin. Everyone knows that the skin of your face and neck must be treated differently than that of the rest of you body.

Our faces are exposed to the elements more than any other area of skin. Irritants are intentionally applied to the face that can cause blemishes and aging if not removed properly. Perhaps most important reason for treating the skin of our face differently is that the facial area is the very first part of your skin most people will notice.

Facial care is one of the best places you can spend time experimenting and customizing to suit your needs. The better customized your facial regimen is to your particular skin type, lifestyle, and needs the better your overall appearance will be. Regardless of the recipes you choose to try it is always recommended that you test sample the products on a sensitive area such as your wrist to ensure you have no unexpected reactions before applying them to your face. This is not a fail proof method of ensuring that the products are correct for you but it can often provide a warning of a negative reaction.

Gentle Scrub for All Skin Types - **foaming**

I love foaming facial washes. The foaming action helps clean the skin and makes application a breeze. This is a favorite cleaner of mine since it is gentle enough for year round use and the natural Vitamins help to improve the look and texture of my skin. This recipe does require refrigeration. Strawberries are rich in Vitamin A & C and have a Ph that is similar to that of our skin. This is an excellent cleanser that nourishes while restoring the natural Ph and providing a natural, healthy glow.

- ➢ 6   Whole Strawberries
- ➢ 2 tbsp.   Hemp Seed Oil
- ➢ 3 tbsp.   Witch Hazel

Blend all ingredients in a blender or food processor until smooth.

- ➢ 1 tbsp.   Almond Oil
- ➢   Emulsifier & Thickener as desired

Gently stir the coconut oil into the mixture until well blended.

Do not whip as the coconut oil will foam.

This recipe has a lovely sweet smell and a pretty pink color but if you desire a specific color or fragrance you may add your favorite colorant or essential oils or herbs to the mixture.

Spoon mixture into a clean container and seal tightly.

Store in the refrigerator for longer shelf life

To use place a small amount in the palm of your hand.

Mix with water. Scrub your face in a gently upward motion.

Basic Cleanser Base - All Skin Types

This is a nice basic cleanser that is effective for all skin types. Oatmeal is great component regardless of your skin needs since it provides gentle cleansing action removing surface dirt and oils without the harsh effects of some other cleansers. I like to add my favorite oils & cleaning products to customize the base for a specific skin need. You can use the mixture as written or refer to the appendix for ingredient ideas.

- 1 cup   Warm Water

- ½ cup   Uncooked Oatmeal

- 1 tbsp.   Glycerin

- 2 drops   Tincture of Benozoin

- Emulsifier & Thickener as desired

Place all of the ingredients in a blender or food processor.

Mix until a pasty texture has been achieved approximately 1-2 minutes.

If you desire a specific color or fragrance you may add your favorite colorant or essential oils or herbs to the mixture.

Store in a tightly sealed container

To apply, place a small amount into the palm of your hand.

Massage into face and skin in an upward motion.

Rinse well and pat dry.

This is a gentle cleanser that works well for all skin types. This mixture may be used on the face and body.

Experiment adding specialized ingredients to suit your skin needs

Replace the water with another liquid agent.

For a foaming effect 2 tbsp. coconut oil may be added to the recipe.

Daily Clarifying Facial for Dry Skin Care

My skin is normal to dry so I don't need much in the way of clarifying washes or rinses, but sometimes during the summer months my skin can get an oily build-up. I like to use this anytime my skin is beginning to look dull for a great clarifying effect.

- ½ cup — Aloe Vera Gel
- 1 tbsp. — Almond Oil
- 3 tbsp. — Witch Hazel
- ¼ tsp. — Tincture of Benzoin
- 1 tbsp. — Coconut Oil
- Emulsifier & Thickener as desired

Mix ingredients in a blender or food processor until well blended.

Approximately 1-2 minutes.

If you desire a specific color or fragrance you may add your favorite colorant or essential oils or herbs to the mixture.

Store in a tightly sealed container

To use massage a small amount into your skin using an upward motion.

Let sit on the skin 30 – 60 seconds

Rinse and pat dry

Daily Foaming Facial Cleanser with Toning Agents

I love the foaming action in my facial cleansers. This is a great recipe for slightly dry when you need a light anti-aging or toning effect. This cleanser provides a moisturizing balm that helps heal damaged skin while giving a light toning action. I modify the recipe by adding ingredients from the alternate ingredient list throughout the year to get the most beneficial results for each season. You can use this cleanser alone or add additional ingredients from the list to ensure the best results for your skin type.

- ➢ 2 tbsp.   Castile Soap
- ➢ 3 tsp.   Honey
- ➢ ¼ cup   Witch Hazel
- ➢ 1 tsp .   Borax Powder
- ➢ 1 tbsp.   Carrot Oil
- ➢ 1 tbsp.   Coconut Oil
- ➢   Emulsifier & Thickener as desired

Stir ingredients (do not beat) until well blended.

If you desire a specific color or fragrance you may add your favorite colorant or essential oils or herbs to the mixture.

Store in a tightly sealed container – pump bottles work well with this base

Toning Cleanser

This cleanser works well at combating dry skin while providing a gentle toning action. The yogurt infuses moisture into the skin while the lemon juice helps restore the skins natural acid levels.

- ½ cup   Unflavored Yogurt

- 1 tbsp   Light Oil-Choose the one you like best

                 I prefer jojoba or safflower

- 2 tsp   Lemon Juice

-      Emulsifier & Thickener as desired

Whip all ingredients until well blended.

Place extra in the refrigerator

To use pour a small amount in the palm of your hand

Massage gently into the skin using an upward motion

Rinse well and pat dry

Moisturizing Cleansing Soap

My skin sometimes gets extra dry in both the summer and the winter causing my skin to appear red and dry. This is a great moisturizing cleanser I like to use anytime I spend a lot of time exposed to the weather. This is a slightly more oily cleanser.

- 1 tsp.   Borax Powder

- ¼ cup   Almond Oil

- ¼ cup   Aloe Vera Gel

- 3 tbsp.   Water

- 2 tbsp.   Apricot Kernel Oil

- Emulsifier & Thickener as desired

Dissolve borax powder in water.

Mix with remaining ingredients until a creamy gel has formed.

If you desire a specific color or fragrance you may add your favorite colorant or essential oils or herbs to the mixture.

Store in a tightly sealed container

Damaged Skin Cleansing Gel

This is an excellent cleansing gel for both the face and body. We use whenever our skin gets sunburned, irritated, or we just need a bit of skin help. The arrowroot powder helps to condition the skin aiding it in retaining moisture and promotes skin healing while the glycerin attracts moisture promoting repair to the damaged skin.

- ➢ 2 tbsp.   Arrowroot Powder

- ➢ 2 tbsp.   Glycerin

- ➢ ¼ cup   Water

- ➢ 1 tsp.   Shea Butter

- ➢   Emulsifier & Thickener as desired

Dissolve powders in water.

Heat the powder and water mixture, stirring frequently until the mixture thickens.

I like to use a double boiler for this process.

If mixture becomes thicker than desired you may add additional water until the desired consistency is obtained.

Mix glycerin into the solution stirring gently until well blended.

I typically do not add color or fragrance to any product designed for damaged skin because additives can cause the irritation to worsen.

If you desire a specific color or fragrance you may add your favorite colorant or essential oils or herbs to the mixture.

Daily Cleanser for Oily Skin

This cleanser is mildly astringent and the juices and honey help clarify oily skin while repairing damages and aiding in the prevention of skin blemishes. This is a great wash I created when we were teenagers and always looking for an effective cleanser to aid in clearing skin eruptions.

- ➢ 1 tsp.   Borax powder
- ➢ ¼ cup   Water

Heat borax and water in a microwave safe dish until just boiling

Approximately 1 minute.

- ➢ 2 tbsp.   Grapefruit juice
- ➢ 2 tsp.   Camphor
- ➢ 1 tsp.   Carrot Oil
- ➢ 1 tsp.   Geranium
- ➢   Emulsifier & Thickener as desired

Add juices and oils to the borax mixture and stir until well blended.

This mixture will be slightly looser than the others so you may wish to add a thickening agent for easier application.

This recipe has a lovely sweet smell and a pretty color but if you desire a specific color or fragrance you may add your favorite colorant or essential oils or herbs to the mixture.

Pour the mixture into a clean container and seal tightly. To apply pour a small amount into the palm of your hand and gently massage into the face with upward motions. Rinse skin and pat dry.

Beauty Milk Cleanser

Milk has long been considered a beauty treatment. This cleanser is excellent for dry to normal skin infusing the skin with moisture while aiding in the restoration of the skins natural Ph. The wash helps improve both the texture and appearance of the skin.

- ➤ ¼ cup   Dry Milk Powder

- ➤ 2 tbsp.   Rosewater

- ➤ 2 tbsp.   Almond Oil

- ➤ 2 tsp.   Lemon Juice

- ➤   Emulsifier & Thickener as desired

Place all ingredients in a blender and blend until a thick paste is formed.

If the finished mixture is too thick you may add regular water until the desired consistency is obtained.

If you desire a specific color or fragrance you may add your favorite colorant or essential oils or herbs to the mixture

The resulting mixture will be a thick paste.

Spoon the mixture into a clean container and seal tightly.

Refrigeration may lengthen the shelf life of the product.

To use, place a small amount of the paste in the palm of your hand and add water.

Apply the resulting mixture in an upward motion into your skin.

Rinse and pat dry

Sweet Radiance Cleanser

This is a lovely gentle cleanser that leaves behind a well hydrated, radiant glow. I love to use this one whenever I need a refreshed look.

> - 2 tbsp   Plain Yogurt

> - 1 tsp   Honey – clover honey works best

> - 2 tbsp   Carrot Oil

> - 1 tbsp   Witch Hazel

> -   Emulsifier & Thickener as desired

Place all ingredients in a blender and blend until a thick paste is formed.

If the finished mixture is too thick you may add regular water or a bit more witch hazel until the desired consistency is obtained.

This cleanser has a beautiful, light fragrance of its own, but If you desire a specific color or fragrance you may add your favorite colorant or essential oils or herbs to the mixture

Spoon the mixture into a clean container and seal tightly.

Refrigeration may lengthen the shelf life of the product. This recipe makes one or two applications. If you choose to enlarge the recipe, refrigeration is a must.

To use, place a small amount of the paste in the palm of your hand.

Apply in an upward motion into your skin.

Rinse and pat dry

Skin Smoothing Cleanser

This is an excellent cleaner I like to use in the winter months when my skin can begin to look dull and blotchy. This is an excellent healing cleanser that helps tighten and tone my skin while improving the texture.

- ½ cup   Aloe Vera Gel

- 1 tbsp.   Powdered Milk

- ¼ cup   Witch Hazel

- 2 tbsp.   Jojoba Oil

-                     Emulsifier & Thickener as desired

Mix all of the ingredients in a blender until a gel has formed.

The mixture will be looser than some of the other cleansers and works very well in a pump.

If you desire a specific color or fragrance you may add your favorite colorant or essential oils or herbs to the mixture

To use apply a small amount to your skin massaging in an upward motion.

Rinse and pat dry

Acne Skin Wash

This wash helps to offset acne eruptions while fading the scarring associated with acne.

- ➢ 1 tsp   burdock root

- ➢ 1/2 cup   hot water

Steep for 30 minutes. Add

- ➢ ½ cup   witch hazel

- ➢ 2 tsp   aloe vera gel

- ➢ 2 tsp   calendula oil

- ➢ 1 tsp   cedarwood oil

- ➢   Emulsifier & Thickener as desired

Pour into a clean, dry bottle with a tight fitting lid

Shake well

Apply to skin with a cotton ball as an astringent wash

3 x's daily

Mixture will separate if left standing. Shake well before use.

Do not use if you are on blood thinning medication, anti-coagulants or have a disorder related to blood
Do not use if you are pregnant or nursing
Do not use if you are unable to use aspirin
Not for use on children
For EXTERNAL use only

At times the skin will require an abrasive action to effectively clean and exfoliate. Exfoliation is the act of lightly abrading the skin to help remove dead skin cells and reveal new skin cells. Because my skin is normal to dry I use exfoliation cleansers only a few times a week because some can be harsher. These can be used daily as desired.

Daily Foaming Facial Scrub for all skin types

This is a great basic recipe for a facial scrub base. I have included the basic options you may use to customize the recipe to your skin type.

The base can be further modified to suit your skin by choosing alternate ingredients from the list included later in the book.

I like this cleanser because it contains more abrasive ingredients and aids in exfoliation. I try to use this cleanser once or twice a week to help reveal better looking skin and improve my skins overall texture.

- ➢ 1 tbsp.   Scrubbing Agent

    Ground Almonds (rougher skin)

    Oatmeal or Cornmeal (gentle cleansing)

    Ground Citrus Peels (clarifying)

- ➢ 1 tbsp.   Coconut Oil

- ➢ 1 tsp.   Honey

- ➢   Emulsifier & Thickener as desired

Toning Facial Scrub

This is another great mildly abrasive scrub that works well as a toning scrub. My mother likes to use this a few times a week to help exfoliate her skin while achieving a younger, more toned look and feel.

- ➤ ½   Chopped Cucumber Peel and Cucumber ground medium fine

- ➤ ¼ cup   Apricot Kernel Oil

- ➤ 2 tbsp.   Cucumber Juice

- ➤ 1 tsp.   Coconut Oil

- ➤ 1 tbsp.   Orange Flower Water

- ➤   Emulsifier & Thickener as desired

Mix all ingredients until well blended.

Stir, do not whip since the coconut oil may foam if whipped.

This recipe has a fresh clean smell and a light color but if you desire a specific color or fragrance you may add your favorite colorant or essential oils or herbs to the mixture.

Daily Clarifying Cleanser for Oily Skin

This cleanser works well for oily skin and is a slightly more soothing alternative to some of the other oily skin options included. I like the light abrasion effect of the oatmeal. I use this cleanser on my body during the summer when sunscreen and oils tend to make my skin a little oilier.

- ¼ cup   Cornstarch
- ¼ cup   Oatmeal
- 2 tbsp   Witch Hazel
- 2 tbsp   Lemon Juice
- 1 tsp   Lavender Oil
- 2 tbsp   Grapefruit Juice
-       Emulsifier & Thickener as desired

Place all ingredients in the blender and whip until the oatmeal is finer and the ingredients are well blended.

The cleaner will have a nice scent from the apples if you desire a specific color or fragrance you may add your favorite colorant or essential oils or herbs to the mixture.

Spoon the cleanser into a clean container and seal tightly.

Store in the refrigerator to extend the shelf life of the product

To use scoop a small amount into your hands and massage into your skin with gentle upward motions

Rinse and pat dry

Blackhead Facial Scrub

My brother suffers from terrible blackheads. I created this facial scrub for him to use on a daily basis. Used in combination with the correct toner and the blackhead treatment stick this has provided dramatic results for him. This is a very loose and liquid form cleanser and may be more difficult to apply.

- ½ Small Tomato

- ¼ cup Cucumber Juice

- 1 tsp. Lemon Juice

- 2 tsp. Witch Hazel

- Emulsifier & Thickener as desired

Combine all ingredients in a blender and blend until well mixed.

This recipe will have a pretty reddish color and a cleaner scent. I typically do not add additional colorants or fragrances to the recipe because the additives may prove more irritating to the skin. If you desire a specific color or fragrance you may add your favorite colorant or essential oils or herbs to the mixture.

Pour into a clean container and seal tightly.

Store in the refrigerator

CHAPTER 3

Astringents & Toners

Astringents & Toners are an essential element in maintaining healthy skin. They work with your cleansers and scrub to help to keep the surface of the skin free of dirt and oils. The cleaner your skin is, the better it absorbs and retains moisture.

Astringents and toners also help to minimize the appearance of pores. You should select astringent and toner recipes that complement your other daily care regimen components. I like to use some of the toners in this recipe throughout the day to keep my skin looking and feeling fresh.

Pippen

BASIC ASTRINGENT

This is a great basic astringent for every day needs and an excellent base for custom astringent products.

> 5 tbsp   Rosewater

You may substitute distilled water if preferred

> 1 tbsp   Witch Hazel

> 1/8 tsp   Borax Powder

Dissolve borax in the rosewater.

You may need to heat the water slightly to help dissolve the borax powder.

Add the vodka and stir well.

Store in an airtight container to prevent evaporation.

Juicy Juice Astringent

Juices from apples, cherries, plums or berries contain sorbitol. Sorbitol is a natural humectant that attracts moisture and provides a smooth texture. This is one of my favorite astringent products because it helps keep my skin fresh while promoting a nice smooth, tight texture.

- ½ cup   Juice of Choice

- 3 tbsp   Rosewater

- 3 tbsp   Witch Hazel

Blend all of the ingredients.

Store an airtight container to prevent evaporation.

Apply to skin using a spritzer bottle or cotton ball.

Wake Up Toner

Whether it is my whole body or just my skin that needs a little wakening, this toner helps speed the processes up! It is easy to make and a perfect choice when we travel.

- 2 tsp   Mint Tea   (two teabags is a good substitute)

- 1 cup   Distilled Water

- ½ cup   Witch Hazel

Steep the tea in the water until you achieve a nice dark brew.

Stir in the witch hazel.

Pour into your favorite spray or dispenser bottle.

Apply to skin using a cotton ball or spritzer.

Do not rinse.

Gentle Astringent for Sensitive Skin

I like this astringent in the winter or whenever my skin is dryer than normal. The liquids are not as drying as pure alcohol but give a wonderfully fresh, toned look to the skin.

> ➢ 4 tbsp   Witch Hazel

> ➢ 4 tbsp   Rosewater

> ➢ 4 tbsp   Orange Flower Water

Blend all of the ingredients in a spray bottle.

Shake well before using.

Cooling Toner

Cucumber juice is one of my favorite astringent products. It helps relieve sore and tired eyes and makes the skin feel refreshingly cool. I love to use this toner when life gets very busy and I need a nice pick me up.

> ➢ ½ cup   Cucumber Juice

> ➢ 4 tbsp   Witch Hazel

> ➢ 2 tbsp   Rosewater

Blend all ingredients and store in an airtight container.

You can make cucumber juice by chopping up one whole cucumber, including the peel. Place it into the blender and whip. Strain off the green juice for use in the recipe.

To apply to eyes, soak cotton balls in the mixture and place over eyes for 10-15 minutes.

To use as an astringent, apply a small amount to your face and neck using a cotton ball or make up removing pad.

Healing Toner

Honey is one of my favorite skin care ingredients. It not only helps to soften the skin, it has antibacterial and healing properties. I make this toner for every teen in the family and for myself whenever my skin gets irritated.

- ➢ 2 tbsp   Honey

- ➢ 4 tbsp   Strong Chamomile Tea

- ➢ 4 tbsp   Rosewater

Blend all of the ingredients and store in an airtight container.

The toner will be sticky at first. Aging helps diminish the sticky quality. I like to age this toner about 1 week before use but you can use it immediately if desired.

Restorative Toner

Sometimes my skin gets irritated. Whether from the wind and sun, an environmental factor, or just from life, I love to use this restorative toner after my wash and mask to help give my skin a little boost on its way to good health.

- ➢ 1 tsp   Honey

- ➢ 1 tsp   Finely Ground Immortelle

- ➢ ¼ cup Aloe Vera Gel

- ➢ ¼ cup Witch Hazel

Blend all of the ingredients and store in an airtight container.

The toner will be sticky at first. Aging helps diminish the sticky quality. I like to age this toner about 1 week before use but you can use it immediately if desired.

Acne Reducing Toner

Acne can be a devastating condition for your skin. Treating acne early and treating it right is critical to saving the appearance of your future self. This is a toner that I like to give to every child in the family as they reach puberty.

- ½ cup   Witch Hazel

- 5 drops   Lemongrass Oil

- 5 drops   Sea Buckthorn Oil

Mix the ingredients in a spritz bottle.

Shake well and spray on affected area 3-4 times a day.

Do not rinse.

CHAPTER 4

Lip Care

Many people forget that proper care of their lips is a vital part of the beauty regimen. Often lipsticks or lip treatments are chosen based upon the color or staying power of the item rather than the content. Lips can age and become unattractive unless proper care is taken to maintain a healthy and youthful appearance.

An important point to remember is that unlike the rest of your skin, lips do not contain any oil glands. This makes it especially important to use products that infuse the lips with moisture while providing a protective coating to prevent drying.

Making lip care products is a very simple process. Often combining only one or two ingredients can make a fantastic product customized toward your skin type and lip care needs. Most people hesitate to create their own lip care products because of their inability to obtain just the right color. There are many natural dye products that can be used to create the perfect color for all of your lip products, lipsticks, lip glosses, even chap sticks! In addition to these natural dye products, there are many chemical colorants that can be blended to obtain just the right shade.

Natural Lip Care Product Colorants

Alkanet Root:
Red root derived comes from a tree

Aids in the dying of products.

This is an excellent base for your lipstick colorant as it is a basic red and could be modified to present a brighter shade or darkened through the use of purple-red beet juice or brown-red henna and tea products.

**Beet Powder
Beet Juice:**
A lovely purple red color

Can be altered or adjusted depending on the shade desired.

This is an easily obtained dye that is a by-product of the beets.

This is one of my favorite colorants because the juice gives the product a light sweet flavor.

Carmine:
Red pigment derived from dried cochineal.

This is another excellent base for your lipstick colorant.

It provides a glowing red shade that can be modified to suit your exact color needs by adding other products to obtain a purple or brown cast.

Cranberry Juice
Creates a gentler form of the red glow found in some other dyes and colorants.

Grape Juice
Stains from grape juice are a common concern around the house. Now, by mixing the lovely dark shade of pure grape juice with other desired colors you can obtain a dye that will provide a lovely purple red glow to your lips

This is another of my favorite colorants because all of the flavor of the grapes will be present every time you apply your gloss or lipstick!

Henna   Most people are unaware that henna powder comes in a variety of shades and that the longer you let the henna soak in the liquid form the darker the shade will become.

This is an excellent colorant for those who desire a darker color or brown red effect.

This color may cause a dyed look to the lips and should be carefully monitored to ensure a semi-permanent lip appearance is not created unless the color is a look you desire.

The use of henna for colorant provides the added benefit of a lip protection ingredient. Henna forms a protective coating which is excellent for the maintenance of your lip condition during harsh climatic conditions.

Tea   For those who prefer a tan or brown shade to their lipstick the addition of tea can provide a lovely color ranging from a light golden glow found in chamomile to a darker brown shade using teas such as orange pekoe.

Experiment with the various teas you currently use paying close attention to the color of the water. To create stronger tones simply steep your tea in a smaller amount of water for longer periods.

The liquid colorants can be used in place of many of the liquids in the following recipes to generate the color you desire.

In addition to color, creating your own lip care products provides another exceptional opportunity for customization. Most people have specific flavorings that they prefer and benefits they require. By creating your own lip care products you have the opportunity to add flavorings that suit you likes and moods.

Moisture Infusing Lip Stick

A good moisturizing lip stick is an essential part of any beauty care regimen. Most of us don't realize how much moisture our lips lose on a daily basis or even that moisture is essential to healthy lips making a moisture infusing stick a must have rather than a beauty extra. This is a nice stick I like to carry with me at all times. I apply a little whenever my lips feel a bit dry. In addition to providing a fantastic protective moisturizer for my lips it looks great!

- ¼ cup   Grated Beeswax

- 1 tbsp.   Lanolin

- 1 tsp.   Petroleum Jelly

- 1 tbsp.   Apricot Kernel Oil

- 2 tbsp.   Favorite Juice

- Flavors, Colors, Emulsifier & Thickener as desired

Pear/apple/cherry/berry juices all provide a moisture attraction. Choose the color juice that is best for your needs.

Additional dyes may be added to alter the color of the stick or the juice may be left out if preferred.

The juice will also provide a pleasant flavoring without the need for additional additives.

Place the grated beeswax, lanolin and petroleum jelly in a microwave safe dish and microwave on medium for approximately 45 seconds.

Remove the mixture from the microwave and allow to cool slightly.

Stir in the apricot kernel oil and preferred juice until well mixed.

Pour the solution in a greased container and allow to cool. Approximately 12-16 hours until solution is hardened. Placing the container in the refrigerator may speed the process.

Cut the hardened product into sticks and apply.

Basic Beeswax Lipstick

I like to use beeswax as my lipstick base. Beeswax is gentle, has many healing and anti-bacterial properties, and makes a firm lipstick that holds up well over time.

- ¼ cup   Grated Beeswax

- 3 tbsp.   Apricot Kernel Oil

- 2 tbsp.   Grated Cocoa Butter

- 1 tbsp.   Coconut Oil

- 2 tbsp.   Lecithin

- 1   Vitamin C Tablet

-                 Flavors, Colors, Emulsifier & Thickener as desired

Mix oils, beeswax and cocoa butter in microwave safe dish.

Microwave on medium approximately 1 minute

When mixture is a golden brown liquid, add the crushed Vitamin C tablet and stir until dissolved.

Allow mixture to cool slightly and stir in your favorite colorant and flavorings as desired. These are not a necessary additive to the mixture.

Pour mixture into a greased container and allow to cool and harden. Approximately 12-16 hours. Placing the container in the refrigerator may speed the process.

Cut the hardened mixture into sticks and apply.

Makes approximately 5 ¼ inch x 2 inch sticks

Protective Lip Stick

We live a very active outdoor life and there are times in both the summer and winter months when my lips need some extra care and attention. This is an excellent basic stick for harsher climates and it works especially well when my lips become chapped. I like to separate the mixture before hardening to add a variety of flavorings and colors.

> 4 tbsp.   Grated Coca Butter   (stick)

> 1 tbsp.   Zinc Oxide

> 1 tsp.   Apricot Kernel Oil

> 1 tsp.   Honey

>   Flavors, Colors, Emulsifier & Thickener as desired

Place grated cocoa butter in a microwave safe dish and microwave on medium heat for approximately 20 seconds until the mixture is a pasty liquid.

Stir in remaining ingredients until well mixed.

Be sure to use only USP Grade for Cosmetic use Zinc Oxide.

Add colorant or flavors as desired.

Pour mixture into a greased container and allow to harden. Approximately 12-16 hours. Mixture may be placed into the refrigerator to speed the process.

Cut mixture into sticks and apply.

These sticks will be slightly softer than the basic lipstick recipe.

Makes approximately 5 ¼ inch x 2 inch sticks

Healing Chapped Lip Stick

This is an especially popular mixture for the guys. Many of the men in my family neglect their lips until they become chapped. Then they want an instant cure. I like to keep a few of these around, especially during the colder months.

- ¼ cup   Grated Beeswax

- 3 tbsp.   Apricot Kernel Oil

- 2 tbsp.   Grated Cocoa Butter

- 1 tbsp.   Aloe Vera Gel

- 1 tsp.   Zinc Oxide

- 1 tsp.   Honey

- Flavors, Colors, Emulsifier & Thickener as desired

Combine all the ingredients in a microwave safe dish.

Use the solid form cocoa butter for best results.

Be sure to use only USP Grade for Cosmetic use Zinc Oxide.

Microwave on medium heat approximately 45 seconds until the mixture is a soft creamy liquid.

Stir gently to combine all ingredients.

Add your favorite colorant or flavorings if desired.

Pour the mixture into a greased container and allow to cool. Approximately 12-16 hours. Placing the container in the refrigerator may speed the cooling process.

Cut the hardened mixture into sticks and apply.

Makes approximately 5 ¼ inch x 2 inch sticks

Almond Oil Lip Gloss

Sometimes a nice glossy look is a must have. When I want a glossy look or just to add some moisture to my lips I use this instead of some of the other products designed to promote healing.

- ➤ 1 tsp.   Grated Beeswax

- ➤ 1 tsp.   Grated Cocoa Butter (stick)

- ➤ 1 tsp.   Almond Oil

- ➤ 1 tsp.   Apricot Kernel Oil

- ➤   Flavors, Colors, Emulsifier & Thickener as desired

Mix all ingredients in a microwave safe dish and microwave on medium heat for approximately 20 seconds.

A thick mixture should form.

Gently stir until all ingredients are well blended.

Add your favorite colorant or flavoring.

Pour into a clean lip gloss container and allow to cool.

Mixture will stay somewhat soft for easy fingertip application.

Moisture Locking Lip Gloss

This is a fantastic finish stick. It gives the lips a nice shiny look and locks in moisture. I like to carry this in my purse for freshening throughout the day.

- ➢ 1 tbsp.   Coconut Oil

- ➢ 1 tbsp.   Petroleum Jelly

- ➢ 1 tbsp.   Apricot Kernel Oil

- ➢ 1 tsp.   Stearic Acid

- ➢   Flavors, Colors, Emulsifier & Thickener as desired

Add favorite colorant or flavoring as desired.

Combine all ingredients in bowl and whip until well mixed approximately 1 minute.

Spoon mixture into lip-gloss container and apply with fingertip or applicator.

For a more liquid from lip-gloss leave out the stearic acid

Liquid can be applied with a brush or sponge applicator.

Thicker Lip Gloss

This recipe creates a much thicker gloss that retains its shine much longer than some of the others. I really love this whenever I know I have hours and hours to go before I can refresh my make up.

> - 10   Psyllium Seeds

> - ½ cup   Boiling Water

Pour boiling water over psyllium seeds and allow to soak for 6-12 hours depending on the thickness desired.

The longer the seeds soak the thicker the final results will become.

Strain liquid from seeds and discard the seeds.

> - ¼ cup   pear juice (apple, cherry, berry)

> - 1   Vitamin C Tablet

> - Flavors, Colors, Emulsifier & Thickener as desired

Crush the Vitamin C tablet and dissolve into the juice mixture.

Slowly add juice mixture to the psyllium seed gel stirring thoroughly.

The mixture will form a very heavy gloss that will provide a high shine and a protective moisturizing base for your lip care.

This gloss is much thicker than usual and you will want to experiment with soak time and the amount of juice added to the seed gel to obtain the best texture for your needs.

The juices you have chosen will provide color, flavor and fragrance to your product, but if you desire a specific color, flavor or fragrance you may add your favorite flavorings, coloring or essential oils to the mixture.

Chapped Lip Balm

Our lips get very chapped when the seasons change. We keep chapped lip balm ready for each member of the family.

- ➢ 10   Alder Leaves

- ➢ ¼ cup   Boiling Water

Pours boiling water over leaves and allow to set for approximately 6 hours until a tea substance is obtained.

- ➢ 1 tsp.   Aloe Vera Gel

- ➢ 3 tbsp.   Petroleum Jelly

- ➢ 3 tbsp.   Stearic Acid

- ➢   Flavors, Colors, Emulsifier & Thickener as desired

Add alder leaves liquid to the other ingredients stirring gently.

The result will be a very soft balm, which can be rubbed into lips for relief from cracking and irritation.

For a thicker end result use more stearic acid and for a softer result use less stearic acid.

Add desired colors or flavorings.

Spoon into a clean gloss container and seal tightly.

To apply use fingertip or applicator to apply a light coat to your lips

Lip Blemish Sticks

At times we all get a pimple, ulcer or other blemish around our lip area. This is an excellent product that will help promote faster healing of these eruptions while aiding in the prevention of additional blemishes.

- ➤ 4 tbsp.   Grated Beeswax

- ➤ 1 tsp.   Honey

- ➤ 2 tbsp.   Apricot Kernel Oil

- ➤ 1 tsp.   Powdered Bloodwort

- ➤ 1   Vitamin C Tablet

- ➤   Flavors, Colors, Emulsifier & Thickener as desired

Place beeswax, honey and oil in a microwave safe dish and heat on medium approximately 25 seconds.

Dissolve powdered bloodwort and crushed Vitamin C tablet in the heated solution and mix well.

If you desire a specific color, flavor or fragrance you may add your favorite flavorings, coloring or essential oils to the mixture.

Pour the mixture into a greased pan and allow to harden approximately 12-16 hours. You may place the container in the refrigerator for faster results.

Cut the hardened mixture into sticks and apply as needed.

CHAPTER
5

Eye Treatments

The skin around your eyes is especially sensitive. While many of the lotions and creams in this guide are suitable for any area of skin, you may want to consider specialized products to help protect the delicate eye area.

There are also a few special problems that can arise with the skin around the eyes. I have included some recipes that will aid you in treating these problems and the ingredient list provides numerous beneficial ingredients that you can use to customize the cleansers, lotions, and serums included elsewhere in this guide to eye care products.

I often make my eye care treatments with very simple, oil based recipes. This helps me to avoid any inadvertent negative side effects that might result from some of the extra ingredients. Each person is different and you may wish to include some of the ingredients from the optional ingredient list. Remember, just because oil based treatments work very well for my eye area, yours may respond better to alternative treatments.

Firming Eye and Neck Cream

This is a wonderful massage for the eye and neck oil, especially before bed. It works wonders all over the face if you skin is exceptionally dry.

- ➢ 2 tsp   Olive Oil

- ➢ 2 tsp   Shea Butter

- ➢ 1 tsp   Apricot Kernel Oil

- ➢ ½ tsp   Vitamin E Oil

- ➢ ½ tsp   Argon Oil

- ➢   Emulsifier & Thickener as desired

Blend all of the oils.

Dab under eyes with fingertips and massage into the neck area.

Do not rinse.

Soothing Eye Firming Gel

My eyes sometimes get a bit puffy but many treatments to reduce puffiness also dry out the sensitive skin at the same time. I love using these oils since they reduce the puffiness while tightening and firming the skin.

- ➢ 2 tsp   Tamanu Oil

- ➢ 2 tsp   Sunflower Oil

Blend oils and apply under eyes and on lids in the morning and at bedtime.

Do not rinse.

Eye Serum

Jojoba is an excellent base for eye creams and serums since it is close to the skins natural oils and easily absorbed. This is my base eye serum for every day use.

- ➢ 2 tsp   Jojoba Oil

- ➢ 2 tsp   Chamomile Oil

- ➢ 1 tsp   Pomegranate

- ➢   Emulsifier & Thickener as desired

Gently blend oils. Store in a pump container that allows you to dispense 1 or 2 drops at a time.

Coco Eye Cream

Coconut oil and coco butter are two of my favorite bases. I like to use them as a base for my nighttime eye cream. This is a firmer cream but not as liquid as a serum. It does not work as well under makeup as some serums but it does tend to stay in place and leave the eyes looking and feeling great when I wake up.

- ➢ 2 tbsp   Shea Butter

- ➢ 2 tbsp   Coconut Oil

- ➢ ½ tsp   Vitamin E Oil

- ➢   Emulsifier & Thickener as desired

Heat the coco butter and coconut oil just enough to soften.

Do not over heat as the Vitamin E Oil can lose many of its beneficial properties if it is exposed to too much heat.

Add the Vitamin E and whip. Store in a plastic or glass jar.

Wrinkle Reducing Serum

This is a wonderful serum that helps to reduce the appearance of fine lines and wrinkles around the eyes.

- ➤ 1 tsp   Jojoba Oil

- ➤ 1 tsp   Argam Oil

- ➤ 1 tsp   Immortelle Oil

- ➤ 2 tsp   Sea Buckthorn Oil

- ➤   Emulsifier & Thickener as desired

Blend all of the oils in your favorite glass or jar. Apply to eye area daily.

Toning Eye Gel

This is a nice toning gel that helps reduce puffiness, plump the skin and sooth tired eyes all at once. This can be too much for those with especially sensitive skin so do a skin test before use.

- ➤ 1 tbsp   Aloe Vera Gel

- ➤ 1 tbsp   Fresh Cucumber juice

- ➤ 1 tbsp   Witch Hazel

- ➤   Emulsifier & Thickener as desired

Heat the aloe and cumber juice about 30 seconds on the microwaves high setting.

Remove from heat and add the Witch Hazel. Stir well. The mixture will thicken as it cools

Spoon into an airtight container.

To use, dab a small amount under each eye

CHAPTER

6

Lotions and Creams

Once you have clean and healthy looking skin and have treated your problem patches, the next important focus to obtaining healthy skin is moisture. Your skin needs moisture to look its best. The basic ingredients in moisturizing products are oil and water. Most creams also contain an emulsifier.

An emulsifier is a waxy substance that aids in keeping oil and water from separating. If you choose not to use an emulsifier the creams and lotions you create will provide the same benefits but the components may separate when the product is left to sit. To correct this separation, shake the skin care product well before applying. This will serve to combine the ingredients and is an effective solution if you don't want an emulsifier in your mixture.

Before you decide which recipes are right for you, you must determine what type of skin you have. There are four basic types of skin: normal, dry, oily, and combination.

Dry skin does not occur when skin is deprived of oils, but rather when water is lacking in the skin. This means that for those of us with dry skin hydrating the skin from the inside as well as the out can go a long way toward curing our most basic skin problems. Dry skin can become very irritated and unattractive.

Proper care and hydration can cure the most common and basic dry skin problems. If you have allowed the problem to become excessive or if you suffer from a specific skin disorder it is best to seek the input of your dermatologist before trying any self-created products as some skin disorders can actually be aggravated by the use of the wrong product.

Oily skin is a surplus of oil on the surface of the skin as well as a build up of oils below the surface which can result in unsightly eruptions and irritation. You will want to limit the amount of oils you utilize if your skin tends towards oily. Your skin has the ability to generate enough oils on its own and one of the focuses of your regimen will be to nourish and care for your skin while limiting the amount of external oil you apply.

There is a very simple method of determining your skin type. Wash your face with your favorite basic cleanser. Pat your skin dry and do not apply any further products to your skin. After a couple of hours take a clean cloth or tissue paper and blot your forehead, nose and cheeks. Using a new cloth for each area of the skin blotted. If oily spots appear on the cloth your skin could be considered oil. If there is only a small amount of oil on the cloths your skin is probably normal. If no oil appears on any of the cloths your skin is likely dry. Skin can change for a variety of reasons: aging changes the oil levels in your skin as do climatic conditions and hormone levels. You may want to test your skin during a variety of conditions to determine what products may benefit you the most during what times of the month or year.

These recipes are ones that I use for face and body lotions and creams. You should consider which ones will best suit your facial and body care needs and then choose the lotions that will work best for you.

Protective Lotion

This is a nice lotion that provides extra skin protection ingredients. I like to use this whenever I will be working outdoors or with chemicals and products that can effect my skin. The beeswax and oils form a protective layer on the skin making it difficult for dirt and harmful chemicals to damage the skin. This is a great lotion year round for normal to dry skin.

- 2 tbsp.   Grated Beeswax

- ¼ tsp.   Borax Powder

- ¼ cup   Apricot Kernel Oil

- ¼ cup   Tincture of Benzoin

- ¼ cup   Water

- Emulsifier & Thickener as desired

Mix the beeswax and oils in a microwave safe dish.

Microwave on medium heat until the beeswax is melted to a syrup consistency – approximately 30 seconds.

Remove the mixture from the microwave and set aside.

Dissolve the borax powder in the water and heat in the microwave until just boiling – approximately 1 minute.

Slowly pour the borax solution into the oil and beeswax mixture.

Whip the mixture with a whisk or in a blender until the mixture foams slightly and all ingredients are well blended.

If you desire a specific color or fragrance for you lotion, add the food coloring or essential oils before blending.

Pour the lotion into a clean container and allow to cool. The lotion will thicken as it cools.

Glowing Daily Lotion

There are currently many products on the market that provide an unnatural glow to the skin. These products contain everything from crystals to metal. This is a fantastic lotion that will allow your skins natural glow to shin through. I love to use this lotion in the summer months when my skin needs nourishment and I can show off the natural glow that is a part of my skin.

> 2 tbsp.   Grated Beeswax

> 1 tbsp.   Lanolin Oil

Heat the beeswax and lanolin in the microwave until they melt to a thick syrup. Approximately 25 seconds.

Heat watermelon Juice and Borax Powder on medium heat in microwave until almost boiling - Approximately 45 seconds.

> ¼ cup   Watermelon Juice

> ¼ tsp. Borax Powder

Slowly add the borax mixture to the beeswax syrup.

> ¼ cup   Aloe Vera Gel

> Emulsifier & Thickener as desired

Add the aloe vera gel and blend ingredients until they are well mixed.

If you desire a special color or fragrance for your lotion add the food coloring or essential oils to the mixture and stir until evenly distributed.

Pour the lotion into a clean container and allow to cool completely.

The mixture will thicken as it stands. Tightly seal the container.

This lotion will not keep as long as some others because of the juice and may be stored in the refrigerator to lengthen the shelf life.

To apply massage a small amount into your skin.

Papaya Rough Skin Lotion

This is an excellent lotion for extremely rough skin patches. Papaya fruit is very rich in papain which is a natural skin softener. This oil rich cream is easily absorbed by your skin aiding in the healing and repair of extremely damaged and rough skin areas. This cream should be stored in the refrigerator to ensure a longer shelf life.

> ➢ 1 medium papaya fruit (unripe fruits contain the highest level of papain)

> ➢ 1 tbsp.   Lecithin

> ➢ 1 tsp.   Baking soda

> ➢ 3 tbsp.   Stearic Acid Powder

> ➢ ¼ cup   Wheat Germ Oil

> ➢   Emulsifier & Thickener as desired

Mix oil, stearic acid and lecithin in a microwave safe dish.

Heat on medium heat until a syrupy foam is formed.

While the oil mixture is heating, mash or blend papaya fruit into a creamy mash. I use the blender for this. Mix the baking soda and papaya until well blended.

Heat the papaya mixture in a microwave safe dish until warmed approximately 40 seconds on medium heat in the microwave.

Add the oil mixture to the papaya base, stirring well.

The mixture will foam while you stir and this should not be a cause for concern.

The product will have its own natural scent and color, but if you desire a specific color to suit your needs or an aromatherapy benefit you may add your favorite colorant or essential oils to the recipe.

Pippen

Pear Lotion for Red Blotchy Skin

This is a great treatment to make anytime environmental factors create havoc with your skin. I love the soft scent of the pears, but you could use other fruits that contain sorbitol such as apples, cherries, plums or berries. Sorbitol is a natural humectrant that attracts moisture and provides a smooth texture. If you have a sensitivity to wool products you might want to replace the lanolin in the mixture with an alternate ingredient from the skin care list.

> 2 tbsp.   Grated Beeswax

> 2 tbsp.   Lanolin

> ¼ cup   Sesame Seed Oil

> ¼ cup   Juice (pear, apple, cherry, plum or berry)

> 2 tbsp.   Witch Hazel

> ¼ tsp.   Borax Powder

>   Emulsifier & Thickener as desired

Combine the beeswax, oils and lanolin in a microwave safe dish and heat on medium for approximately 30 seconds until the waxes are melted to a thick syrup.

Combine the juice, witch hazel and borax in another dish.

Heat until mixture is hot but not boiling —approximately 35 seconds on medium heat.

Pour the juice mixture into the oil mixture. Stir well.

I love the natural smells and colors of this recipe and can alter the final product by changing the type of juice I use.

You may desire a specific color or fragrance and my add the food coloring or essential oils to the mixture as it cools, stirring well.

Allow the recipe to cool. The mixture will thicken as it cools.

Basic Body Lotion

I always have a basic body lotion on hand. This is a good, general body lotion for everyday use.

- ➢ ¼ cup   Cocoa Butter (tub or grated stick)

- ➢ 1 tbsp.   Coconut Oil

- ➢ 1 tbsp.   Sesame Seed Oil

- ➢ 1 tbsp.   Apricot Kernel Oil

- ➢ 2 tbsp.   Grated Beeswax

- ➢   Emulsifier & Thickener as desired

Combine all ingredients in a microwave safe dish and heat on medium until cocoa butter and beeswax are melted to a thick syrup. Approximately 35 seconds.

Remove from heat and stir to blend.

Pour into a clean container and allow the mixture to cool slightly.

The product will have its own natural scent and color, but if you desire a specific color to suit your needs or an aromatherapy benefit you may add your favorite colorant or essential oils to the recipe.

Stir as the mixture cools to keep the ingredients blended.

When mixture is cooled completely seal container and apply as desired.

Hydrating/Softening Lotion

- ¼ cup   Almond Oil
- ¼ cup   Stearic Acid Powder
- 1 tbsp.   Liquid Lecithin
- ¼ cup   Pear Juice
- ¼ cup   Carrot Juice
- 1 tsp.   Baking Soda
- 2-3 drops   Tincture of Benzoin
- Emulsifier & Thickener as desired

Mix the oils, stearic acid and lecithin in a microwave safe dish.

Microwave on medium until mixture turns golden and foamy – approximately 35 seconds.

Set oil mixture aside.

Combine remaining ingredients in another dish.

Heat on medium until hot but not boiling – approximately 30 seconds

Combine both mixtures, stirring thoroughly until well blended.

The mixture will foam as you stir.

The product will have its own natural scent and color, but if you desire a specific color to suit your needs or an aromatherapy benefit you may add your favorite colorant or essential oils to the recipe.

Allow mixture to cool and pour into a clean container.

Seal tightly and store in the refrigerator for the longest shelf life.

Apply daily for a soft, well hydrated skin.

Irritated Skin Balm

This is a light, non-greasy balm that helps sooth dry or irritated skin. I sometimes get rashes from things I come in contact with outdoors in the summer. This balm helps sooth any irritation that may occur from outside sources or just from dry skin. I also like using this balm for the babies when they have a diaper rash or other irritation. The ingredients soothe the skin and the lavender oils help calm the nerves.

- ½ cup   Aloe Vera Gel

- ¼ cup   Apple Juice

- 2 tsp.   Cornstarch

- 1 tbsp.   Witch Hazel

- 3 drops   Lavender Oil

- 1 tbsp.   Zinc Oxide

-                 Emulsifier & Thickener as desired

Combine the aloe vera gel, apple juice, zinc and witch hazel in a microwave safe dish.

Stir well

Heat on medium approximately 30 seconds until you have a liquid.

Allow the mixture to cool slightly and add the cornstarch and oil.

The product will have its own natural scent and color, but if you desire a specific color to suit your needs or an aromatherapy benefit you may add your favorite colorant or essential oils to the recipe.

Pour the mixture into a clean container and cool completely. Seal tightly.

This mixture will be a little runnier than some of the other lotions so you may apply as usual or use a cotton ball for easier application.

Massage the mixture into affected area until relief is obtained.

Severe Irritation Balm

When skin irritation is a little more severe, such as the first or second day, I like to use something a little stronger. This balm should not be used on children and you should consult your physician before using any product if a severe irritation is present. Arrowroot is an anti-inflammatory that helps reduce the swelling that is often present with skin irritation while the other ingredients reduce the pain and itchiness. I especially like this balm for problems such as itchy nettles or a contact rash from another source.

- ➢ 1 tbsp.   Chamomile Leaves

- ➢ ½ cup   Boiling Water

Pour the water over the chamomile leaves and let steep at least 6 hours until a darker tea is created.

Strain the leaves from the tea and discard.

- ➢ 1 tbsp.   Arrowroot Powder

- ➢ ¼ tsp. Borax powder

- ➢ 1 tsp.   Baking Soda

Dissolve the powders in the tea solution.

- ➢ 1 tbsp.   Jojoba Oil

- ➢ 1 tbsp. Zinc Oxide

- ➢ 1 tbsp.   Grated Beeswax

- ➢ 1 tbsp.   Sunflower Oil

- ➢   Emulsifier & Thickener as desired

Heat oil, zinc and beeswax in a microwave safe dish until a thicker syrup is formed.

Slowly pour the tea mixture into the oil mixture. Whip or use a blender to combine the ingredients.

Deep Moisturizing Cream

This is a deep penetrating cream that I use all over but truly love after a rough skin exfoliation. Beyond the penetration the treatment leaves a protective film on the skin that helps prevent drying due to harsh climatic conditions. My mother makes a heat pack out of this during the winter months, applying a thicker layer of the cream and then covering her hands and feet in plastic to let the oils really penetrate her skin.

- ½ cup   Sesame Oil

- ¼ cup   Wheat Germ Oil

- 2 tbsp.   Grated Beeswax

- 2 tbsp.   Coconut Oil

- Emulsifier & Thickener as desired

Combine oils and beeswax in a microwave safe dish. Heat until a thick syrup is formed approximately 35 seconds.

Allow mixture to cool stirring occasionally.

The product will have its own natural scent and color, but if you desire a specific color to suit your needs or an aromatherapy benefit you may add your favorite colorant or essential oils to the recipe.

Spoon into a clean container and seal tightly.

Apply directly to the desired area and massage gently.

For a deeper condition, heat the mixture slightly under warm water and apply a thick coat to desired areas.

Cover the areas with saran wrap or a plastic bag and allow the mixture to penetrate the skin for 10-15 minutes.

Wipe remaining lotion from skin, do not rinse.

Summer Nourishing Lotion

This is a great nourishing lotion that contains many essential Vitamins that are Vital for healthy skin. This treatment also contains a natural PH much like skin so it aids in restoring skins natural Ph Levels and provides a great lotion for all skin types.

- ½ cup   Almond Oil
- 1 tbsp.   Grated Beeswax
- 1 tbsp.   Liquid Lecithin

Combine oil, lecithin and beeswax in a microwave safe dish and heat on medium until wax melts to a syrup – approximately 45 seconds.

Stir mixture and set aside

- ¼ tsp. Borax Powder
- ½ cup   Water

Heat borax and water in a microwave safe dish until just boiling approximately 45 seconds

Pour borax mixture into beeswax mixture stirring until well blended.

- ¼ cup   Mashed Strawberries

Add the strawberry mash and continue stirring.

You should use a wire whisk and blend quickly or a blender to ensure the ingredients are well mixed.

If you desire a particular color or fragrance you may add your preferred food coloring or essential oils to the mixture and stir well.

Pour the finished product into a clean container and allow to cool completely. Seal tightly and store in the refrigerator.

Massage a small amount of the mixture into your skin as desired.

Moisturizing Staple

This is a good basic moisturizer I keep as a staple in our house. The ingredients work well for all members of the family and the texture is a very light liquid making it an effective moisturizer for all skin types. I like to keep a container of this moisturizer in all the most convenient places, on the sinks, by the computer, anywhere someone might be when they realize they need a little extra moisture.

- ➤ 1 tbsp.   Shea Butter

- ➤ 2 tbsp.   Almond Oil

- ➤ 1 tsp.   Coconut Oil

- ➤ 1 tsp.   Mineral Oil

Combine the lecithin and oils in a microwave safe dish.

Heat in microwave approximately 20 seconds or until coconut oil melts.

Stir gently and set aside.

- ➤ ¼ tsp. Borax Powder

- ➤ ¼ cup   Water

Dissolve borax in the water and heat until just boiling. Approximately 45 seconds in the microwave.

Pour the borax mixture over the oils and stir until well blended.

I like to use a wire whisk to add air to the mixture or a blender.

The product will have its own natural scent and color, but if you desire a specific color to suit your needs or an aromatherapy benefit you may add your favorite colorant or essential oils to the recipe.

The mixture will become smooth and creamy. Pour into a clean container and use as desired.

Lanolin and Aloe Cream

This is a good cream for the winter months when skin can be come dry and chapped. I like to use this mixture anytime my skin needs a little extra protection. Do not use this cream if you have a sensitivity to wool products.

- ½ cup   Aloe Vera Gel

- 3 tbsp.   Lanolin Oil

- 1 ½ tsp.   Corn starch

- ¼ cup   Avocado Oil

- 2 tbsp.   Beeswax

- Emulsifier & Thickener as desired

Combine the oils and beeswax in a microwave safe dish and heat on medium for approximately 35 seconds or until beeswax and lanolin is melted.

Slowly stir in the cornstarch and aloe vera gel until well blended.

The product will have its own natural scent and color, but if you desire a specific color to suit your needs or an aromatherapy benefit you may add your favorite colorant or essential oils to the recipe.

Allow mixture to cool completely.

Spoon into a clean container and seal tightly.

This is a thick cream that works very well for irritated or chapped skin.

To apply massage gently into the affected areas

Acne Topical Ointment

- ¼ cup jojoba oil

- 1 tsp sandalwood oil

- 1 tsp camphor

- 1 tsp adder's tongue

- 1 tsp cypress oil

Apply a thin coat to skin morning and night. Do not rinse. Do not use around eye area.

Do not use if you are on blood thinning medication, anti-coagulants or have a disorder related to blood

Do not use if you are pregnant or nursing

Do not use if you are unable to use aspirin

Not for use on children

For EXTERNAL use only

Skin Smoothing Lotion

This is a lovely light lotion that I like to use year-round. It works especially well in the summer because it provides a great treatment for dry skin that sometimes comes with too much sun exposure. The corn flour provides a silky texture to the lotion that leaves the skin feeling supple and smooth while the natural humectants qualities of the glycerin attract moisture to provide a softening quality.

- 3 tbsp.   Glycerin
- 3 tbsp.   Corn Flour (cornstarch powder)
- ¼ cup   Rosewater
- ¼ cup   Water
- Emulsifier & Thickener as desired

Mix all of the ingredients in a microwave safe dish. Heat 1-2 minutes until the mixture comes to a boil. Stir every 20-25 seconds during heating.

The product will have its own natural scent and color, but if you desire a specific color to suit your needs or an aromatherapy benefit you may add your favorite colorant or essential oils to the recipe.

Allow the lotion to cool completely.

Pour into a clean container and seal tightly.

To use pump or pour a small amount into the palm and massage gently into the skin

This lotion is more gel like than some of the others.

Deep Moisture Infuser

This is a rich lotion that will infuse your skin with moisture. The lotion contains many oils and essential Vitamins that are essential to healthy skin. This is a nice deep moisturizing treatment that is beneficial for the entire body and works wonders on dry, scaly patches.

- 2 tbsp.   Grated Beeswax

- 2 tbsp.   Sesame Oil

- 1 tbsp.   Apricot Kernel Oil

- 1 tbsp.   Avocado Oil

- 1 tsp.   Vitamin E Oil

- 1 tsp.   Wheat Germ Oil

- 1 tsp.   Almond Oil

-                Emulsifier & Thickener as desired

Combine the oils and beeswax in a microwave safe dish.

Heat on medium in the microwave until the mixture forms a thick syrup approximately 40 seconds.

Stir the beeswax and oils. Add

- 1 tsp.   Baking soda

- ¼ cup   Rosewater

Whip ingredients until well blended.

If you desire a specific color or fragrance add food coloring or preferred essential oil to the mixture and stir until evenly distributed.

Allow the mixture to cool completely. Pour into a clean container and seal tightly.

Firming Night Gel

This is a great gel I like to use at night so I can obtain the full benefits. The lotion contains many conditioning oils and aids skin in appearing firm and supple.

- ➤ 1 tbsp.   Coconut Oil

- ➤ 2 tbsp.   Almond Oil

- ➤ 2 tsp.   Avocado Oil

- ➤ 1 tsp.   Vitamin E Oil

- ➤ 1 tbsp.   Apricot Kernel Oil

- ➤ 1 tbsp.   Mineral Oil

- ➤ 2 tbsp.   Aloe Vera Gel

- ➤   Emulsifier & Thickener as desired

Combine all ingredients in a microwave safe dish. Heat on medium in the microwave approximately 50 seconds

Remove from microwave and stir well to blend the ingredients.

If you desire a particular color or fragrance, add the food coloring or the essential oils of your choice and stir well to evenly distribute.

Pour the lotion into a clean container and allow to cool completely.

The lotion will thicken as it cools. Seal tightly and apply a small amount to the skin before bed each night for an effective firming treatment.

Cellulite Reducing Lotion

Other sections of this book have recipes which help reduce the appearance of cellulite and combat the signs of aging. This lotion provides much the same benefits and works great as a daily lotion or in combination with some of the other treatments for special events. The Irish Moss helps remove dead skin cells provide a cleaner, age-defying effect to the skin while the English Ivy draws excess moisture from beneath the surface of the skin reducing puffiness and the appearance of cellulite.

> - 1 tbsp.   Powdered Irish Moss

> - 2 tbsp.   Powdered English Ivy Leaves

> - 1 cup Rosewater

> -   Emulsifier & Thickener as desired

Mix the Irish Moss, Ivy and rosewater in a microwave safe dish and let soak for 20-30 minutes.

After soaking heat the mixture in the microwave until just boiling – approximately 1 ½ minutes

Allow the mixture to soak an additional 10-15 minutes.

Strain the solids from the liquid and discard.

> - 1 cup Aloe Vera Lotion

> - 3 tbsp.   cucumber juice

> - 3 tbsp.   jojoba oil

> - 3 tsp.   Vitamin E oil

Pour the remaining ingredients into your seaweed gel. Whip or blend until well mixed. The product will have its own natural scent and color, but if you desire a specific color to suit your needs or an aromatherapy benefit you may add your favorite colorant or essential oils to the recipe.

Hydrating Daily Lotion

Skin doesn't just need moisture on the surface, skin needs moisture deep down. Hydrating washes, lotions and treatments provide the benefit of total moisture infusion. This lotion is great for daily use to provide a supple, healthy appearance to skin.

- ➤ 2 tbsp.   Dried Chamomile Leaves

- ➤ ½ cup   Boiling Water

Pour the water over the chamomile leaves and allow the mixture to steep for at least 6 hours.

The longer the mixture steeps the stronger the resulting tea will be and the more powerful your lotion will become.

Strain the leaves from your tea solution and discard.

- ➤ 3 tbsp.   Stearic Acid Powder

- ➤ 1 tsp.   Baking Soda

- ➤ 3 tbsp.   Glycerin

- ➤ ¼ cup   Jojoba Oil

- ➤   Emulsifier & Thickener as desired

Combine the baking soda and glycerin with the chamomile water in a microwave safe dish. Heat on medium until the mixture just reaches boiling approximately 1 minute.

Stir gently.

> ➤ ½ cup   Carrot Juice

Add the carrot juice to the chamomile tea mixture and stir gently.

Combine the oils and the stearic acid in a microwave safe dish and heat on medium until the liquid runs clear – approximately 30 seconds.

Slowly pour the chamomile mixture into the oil base.

The mixture will foam as it is mixed.

Stir gently to combine remaining ingredients.

Allow mixture to cool.

The mixture will have a pretty golden orange color and a delicate fragrance. If you desire a personalized fragrance or color you may add food coloring or your favorite essential oils to the mixture as it cools.

Stir well to be sure additives are evenly distributed.

Pour mixture into a clean container and seal tightly.

Massage a small amount into the skin desired daily for a pretty hydrated glow.

Age-Defying Lotion

This is an effective lotion for the body that infuses the skin with various age-defying components. This lotion will aid in the toning of the skin.

- ➤ 1 tbsp.   Fennel Seeds
- ➤ ¼ cup   Boiling Water

Pour the boiling water over the fennel seeds and allow the mixture to soak overnight.

- ➤ 2 tbsp.   Grated Beeswax
- ➤ 1 tbsp.   Lanolin
- ➤ 1 tsp.   Vitamin E oil
- ➤ 1 tbsp.   Wheat Germ Oil

Combine beeswax and oils in a microwave safe dish and heat until melted approximately 45 seconds.

Remove from heat and stir to blend the oils.

- ➤ 2 tbsp. Aluminum Sulfate
- ➤ 3 tbsp. witch hazel
- ➤ 3 tbsp. orange flower water
- ➤   Emulsifier & Thickener as desired

Use only USP Grade for Cosmetic Use aluminum sulfates.

Use only plastic or ceramic pans and utensils as aluminum sulfate can react with metals.

Dissolve the aluminum sulfate in the witch hazel and orange flower water.

Add fennel seed liquid and stir well.

Slowly pour the liquid solution into the oil base stirring well.

The mixture will foam slightly as you stir.

The product will have its own natural scent and color, but if you desire a specific color to suit your needs or an aromatherapy benefit you may add your favorite colorant or essential oils to the recipe.

Allow solution to cool completely.

Spoon into a clean container and seal tightly.

Massage in to the skin of the body and neck twice daily for the most beneficial results.

Lotion to Silkening Powder

Add 2 tablespoons of french talc or another preferred powder to your lotion.

Whip well.

Apply as you would any lotion.

As it dries, it leaves a beautiful silky feeling behind.

This is one of our favorite lotions for hands and feet.

Skin Toning Lotion

At times I want an all over body toning product and don't want to use the toners created specifically for facial care. This is a great lotion that provides a fresh clean feel while delivering toning agents to my skin.

- ➤ 2 tbsp.   Lanolin

- ➤ 3 tbsp.   Liquid Lecithin

- ➤ 2 tbsp.   Wheat Germ Oil

Blend the ingredients in a microwave safe dish and heat until just melted approximately 30 seconds. Stir gently to blend.

- ➤ ¼ cup   Witch Hazel

- ➤ 2 tbsp.   Rosewater

- ➤ ¼ cup   Stearic Acid Powder

- ➤   Emulsifier & Thickener as desired

Dissolve the powder in the witch hazel and rosewater.

Slowly pour the mixed liquid into the oil base stirring well.

The product will have its own natural scent and color, but if you desire a specific color to suit your needs or an aromatherapy benefit you may add your favorite colorant or essential oils to the recipe.

Allow the mixture to cool completely.

The mixture will thicken as it cools.

Pour into a clean container and seal tightly.

Massage into skin for a refreshing feel and well toned appearance.

Soaps

Perhaps the most basic product in your daily personal care ritual is soap. Before you can use any other product in your regimen the area you are treating must be clean. The importance of using the correct soap is often overlooked.

Consider that soap is the first item, and often the last, that you use each day. People often spend the rest of the day using products to counteract the effects of the soap they have chosen. Using the correct soap can either harm or enhance the rest of your products.

Before deciding which soap recipe to try, you should understand the basics of skin and skin care. There are many factors that can effect the condition and appearance of skin. No soap or other product can replace simple daily care in your activities. Skin is the largest organ you have and perhaps the most important in that it protects every other part of you from environmental factors. Of course skin is also very important because it is the first thing most people will notice about you.

Soap is often a very personal decision. People have been creating soaps for generations. The best way to achieve perfection in your soap-making endeavor is to keep experimenting to determine which soap works best with your skin, lifestyle, and climate. This chapter outlines the creation of the most common types of soap that you can customize to suit your needs. I have also included a few of my favorite soap customizations for you to use as a starting point. Remember to experiment – most of the ingredients in soap making are extremely cost effective and easy to locate! You can customize a different soap for each member of your family and then produce these a few times a year for less than you would commonly pay for a decent quality, but generic soap in the stores.

Soap recipes are often the most difficult for most people to follow. Soap requires more time and effort than most of the other products included in this book. Do not be discouraged by the processes described since soap is a common item that has been successfully created by individuals for generations. To create exceptional soaps you will need to practice and perfect your skills. You will also need some slightly different equipment to create soap. You can easily find these items in specialty craft stores or often in an all-in-one retail chain. Some stores even carry kits that contain most of the key equipment in one simple package.

Basic Supplies

Thermometer   Soap making depends heavily on temperature.

The base components such as lye, borax, or even fat must be heated to a particular temperature and then cooled to become soap.

A good method of ensuring the proper temperatures are reached is to obtain a decent candy thermometer.

The thermometer should be used only for one particular type of soap and should be dedicated only to soap making. If you decide to experiment with soaps that have a variety of bases you will want to obtain a few thermometers since using the same thermometer for lye that you use for fat bases can throw off the final results of your soap making endeavor.

Thermometers can be easily found in most craft stores or in the cooking section of your grocery store and need not be the most advanced or expensive model available. A simple, cost-effective thermometer will work just fine for these recipes.

Pot

You will need a glass or steel pot for heating and mixing.

You should have a dedicated mixing container for your soap making endeavors. While most of the ingredients in soap are safe, you would not want to eat out of the same pan you just used for boiling lye.

It is important not to use aluminum or iron pots and pans when creating soap as it can react with the ingredients of the soap. A basic steel or enamel coated pot, which can be found in most retail chain stores works best and is often the most cost-effective purchase.

Wooden Spoons

You will want to purchase a set of wooden utensils for soap making.

Again, these should be dedicated only to your personal care product recipes and not used for cooking.

The kind with longer handles often prove beneficial as you will need to stir deep into your cooking pots to ensure all the ingredients are well mixed.

Wooden utensils work the best as they are heat resistant and will hold up better under some of the stronger ingredients you may choose to use.

Gloves

The final product of your soap making process will be used on your skin, but the core ingredients, before being properly blended, can cause irritation or even burns to the skin. Using a pair of kitchen gloves is the best practice during your soap making. These will protect your hands from inadvertent splashing and prevent problems, which will then need to be treated using a different recipe.

Soap molds

You will need a mold or container to pour your soap in for hardening.

The recipes you will use will often finish as a cake of soap. Caked soap is the most commonly used soap in most households. To achieve these perfectly formed cakes you will need the proper mold. There are many molds available in specialty craft stores as well as retail chains. Soap making has gained popularity in the last few years making these products easier to find than ever before. You can find molds ranging from the very basic cake soap style to the more specialized styles that will suit your décor or even the user of the soap such as children.

You do not need to purchase specialized soap mold. Many common items found in your house will work as well. You can use old baking pans such as muffin pans or even bread pans (you will want to cut the finished soap into bars). You can use cardboard boxes, candy molds (although they will not be suitable for candy making after being used with your soap) almost any container that can withstand the heat and will hold the liquid soap in place while it hardens.

The key to best soap mold use is to be sure that the mold is well oiled and lined with wax paper to keep the cakes of soap from sticking to the mold.

SOAP MAKING DO'S!

Work in a well-ventilated area. Liquid and heated forms of some ingredients included can create fumes, which may be harmful.

Always wear gloves and other protective clothing since lye and other ingredients can burn or irritate the skin.

Always use COLD water when mixing lye solutions.

Pour the lye mixture into the fat mixture not the other way around.

Keep solvents nearby such as vinegar to neutralize the effect of the ingredients if they should come in contact with the skin.

Remember that lye is a poison and should always be kept in a safe place.

Only create heated soap mixtures when you can be sure that you will not be distracted. Some of the ingredients and the heat processes involved in soap making can be dangerous to others who are not prepared. IN addition the recipes included in this chapter require a fine attention to detail to ensure success in your soap-making endeavor.

Tallow Based Soaps

Tallow or fat can be obtained from a variety of sources and has been used for generations in soap making. You can collect clean fat as you cook. Simply trim off clean beef or pork fat before you cook your meat and save it, preferably in the freezer – until you are ready to make soap. Your local butcher or meat department will often provide you with excess fat they have trimmed from their products for free.

➢ Measure your clean fat depending on the quantity of soap you desire.

   One bar of soap will need approximately 1 cup of clean fat.

➢ Place your fat in your soap making container and slowly heat until it is completely melted.

➢ Allow your mixture to cool to approximately 115 degrees Fahrenheit.

➢ You may add borax powder to the melted fat if you desire.

   Use one teaspoon of borax powder per bar of soap being created.

   You do not have to add borax but it does give a better appearance and lather to your soap.

   If you add the borax, stir the powder into your tallow mixture until well blended.

➢ If you desire a specific color or fragrance for your soap you may add your favorite food coloring or essential oils to the mixture.

While your tallow mixture is cooling to the desired temperature you will need to create the lye solution. Again remember that protective gloves and clothing should be worn when using lye because it can burn the skin.

Lye is a poison and unused amounts should be stored in a safe place.

➢ Dissolve the lye granules in cool water.

Approximately 3 teaspoons of lye to ½ cup water for each bar of soap being created.

➤ Once the lye granules are dissolved you will slowly pour the lye mixture into the fat mixture.

Pour in a slow steady stream while stirring the mixture.

You should not have the heat on the mixture at this time.

➤ Stir the ingredients until thick syrup is formed. Approximately 10-20 minutes.

➤ If the soap mixture is not becoming thick after 30 minutes or has a greasy layer floating on the top the mixture may be too warm.

Set the container in a pan of cool water.

Continue stirring being sure to stir the sides and bottom of the pan to ensure an even mix.

➤ If the soap mixture is too lumpy your mixture may be too cold.

If this occurs, reverse the above process.

Sit the mixture in a pan of warm water stirring until the lumps dissolve.

Depending on the consistency you may need to replace your warm water more than once until the mixture is heated to the correct temperature for effective blending.

➤ Once you have obtained the desired texture you may add fragrance or color to suit your desires.

➤ Pour the thickened mixture into your molds and cover.

➤ Keep the mixture in a warm place for at least 2 days.

This helps keep the mixture from separating.

➢ Once the soap has set, remove from the molds and cut into bars if needed.

➢ Place the soap in a dry area to age.

The aging of soap ensures a better quality will be obtained when you use the soap.

You should allow your tallow soap to age at least 2-3 weeks prior to use.

At times you will find that your soap is lumpy or has separated during the aging process. If this occurs do not throw out the failed soap.

➢ Cut the flawed cakes of soap into small pieces – a grater works well for this process.

➢ Return the pieces to your soap making pan and add approximately 1 cup of water for each cake of ground soap.

➢ Dissolve the soap in the water over low heat.

➢ Stir occasionally to ensure the soap does not become overheated.

➢ When the lumps have disappeared and a syrupy texture has been obtained, pour the soap into your favorite molds and follow the process for storage outlined earlier.

This will often cure the problem and provide you with a successful soap.

Glycerin Soap

Another form of cake soap commonly used and sometimes preferred over tallow soap is a glycerin-based soap.

Glycerin is found naturally in many plants and is actually a by-product of the soap making process. When making a fat and lye mixture soap there is often a clear, thick liquid that floats on the top of the mixture. This is glycerin.

Glycerin soap is simply a basic soap to which you add extra glycerin. This soap is excellent for all skin types as it tends to be very mild and glycerin is a natural humectrant that draws and retains moisture in your skin.

To create glycerin you should begin the process is very similar to tallow soap making. The following recipe will make approximately 1 bar of soap and can be enlarged to suit your desired quantity.

➢ Heat 1/3 cup of your favorite vegetable based oil.

Review the oil ingredient list to determine which oil will provide the most beneficial effect for your needs.

Heat the oil to approximately 80 degrees in your soap-making pan.

➢ While your oils are heating dissolve 2 tsp. lye in 1/3 cup cold water.

Remember to wear protective gloves and clothing when working with lye as lye can burn your skin.

Store your unused lye granules in a safe place, as lye is a poison.

➢ Remove your oil mixture from the heat and allow to cool slightly – approximately 70 degrees.

➢ If you desire a specific color or fragrance for your soap you may add your favorite food coloring or essential oils to the mixture.

> ➤ Slowly pour the lye solution into the oil mixture.

> ➤ Stir the mixture gently but mix well to ensure all ingredients are well blended.

> ➤ When the ingredients are well blended add 3 tsp. glycerin.

> ➤ Continue stirring the mixture until well blended.

> ➤ The mixture will take on the consistency of thick syrup.

If the soap mixture does not thicken as desired within 30 minutes or there is a greasy layer on the top of the mixture it may be too warm.

> ➤ Set the container to cool in a pan of cool water.

> ➤ Continue stirring being sure to stir the sides and bottom of the pan to ensure an even mix.

If the soap mixture is too lumpy your mixture may be too cold. If this occurs, reverse the above process.

> ➤ Sit the mixture in a pan of warm water stirring until the lumps dissolve.

> ➤ Depending on the consistency you may need to replace your warm water more than once until the mixture is heated to the correct temperature for effective blending.

Pour the thickened mixture into your molds and cover.

> ➤ Keep the mixture in a warm place for at least 2 days.

  This helps keep the mixture from separating.

Once the soap has set, remove from the molds and cut into bars if needed.

Place the soap in a dry area to age.

> ➤ The aging of soap ensures a better quality will be obtained when you use the soap.

> ➤ You should allow your tallow soap to age at least 2-3 weeks prior to use.

At times you will find that your soap is lumpy or has separated during the aging process. If this occurs do not throw out the failed soap.

> ➤ Cut the flawed cakes of soap into small pieces – a grater works well for this process.

> ➤ Return the pieces to your soap making pan and add approximately 1 cup of water for each cake of ground soap.

> ➤ Dissolve the soap in the water over low heat.

> ➤ Stir occasionally to ensure the soap does not become overheated.

> ➤ When the lumps have disappeared and a syrupy texture has been obtained, pour the soap into your favorite molds and follow the process for storage outlined earlier.

This will often cure the problem and provide you with a successful soap.

Pippen

Beeswax Soap

Beeswax soap is another soap that is gaining in popularity. Creating this soap is sometimes a bit more expensive than the other forms as beeswax is costly in some areas. Check with your health food stores or a beekeeping compound in your area to price beeswax. Beeswax has natural healing and antibacterial properties and will provide a protective coating to the skin. This is one of the better quality soaps for those with sensitive or dry skin.

The process for making beeswax soap is similar to that of the other cake soap recipes contained in the book. The following recipe will make approximately 1 bar of soap and can be enlarged to suit your desired quantity.

> Heat 1/3 cup of your favorite vegetable based oil.

   Review the oil ingredients list to determine which oil will provide the most beneficial effect for your needs.

> Add 4 tsp. grated beeswax to the oils and heat until melted.

   The mixture will be approximately 90 degrees.

> While your oils are heating dissolve 2 tsp. lye in 1/3 cup cold water.

   Remember to wear protective gloves and clothing when working with lye as lye can burn your skin.

   Store your unused lye granules in a safe place since lye is a poison.

> Remove your oil mixture from the heat and allow to cool slightly – approximately 70 degrees.

> If you desire a specific color or fragrance for your soap you may add your favorite food coloring or essential oils to the mixture.

> Slowly pour the lye solution into the oil mixture.

> ➤ Stir the mixture gently but mix well to ensure all ingredients are blended.

If the soap mixture does not thicken as desired within 30 minutes or there is a greasy layer on the top of the mixture it may be too warm.

> ➤ Set the container to cool in a pan of cool water.

> ➤ Continue stirring being sure to stir the sides and bottom of the pan to ensure an even mix.

> ➤ The mixture will become thicker taking on the consistency of thick syrup.

If the soap mixture is too lumpy your mixture may be too cold. If this occurs, reverse the above process.

> ➤ Sit the mixture in a pan of warm water stirring until the lumps dissolve.

> ➤ Depending on the consistency you may need to replace your warm water more than once until the mixture is heated to the correct temperature for effective blending.

Once you have obtained the desired texture you may add fragrance or color to suit your desires.

> ➤ Pour the thickened mixture into your molds and cover.

> ➤ Keep the mixture in a warm place for at least 2 days.

> This helps keep the mixture from separating.

Once the soap has set, remove from the molds and cut into bars if needed.

Place the soap in a dry area until you are ready to use it.

Pippen

coconut Oil Soap

Coconut oil is an excellent skin protectant and is one of the few natural foaming products you can find to use in the soap making process

The following recipe will yield approximately one bar of soap and can be enlarged to suit your desired quantity.

- ➢ Heat 3 tsp. coconut oil and ¼ cup vegetable based shortening on low heat until they reach approximately 75 degrees Fahrenheit.

- ➢ While the mixture is heating dissolve 2 tsp. lye granules in 1/3 cup cold water.

  Remember to wear protective gloves and clothing when working with lye as lye can burn your skin.

  Store your unused lye granules in a safe place, as lye is a poison.

- ➢ Remove your oil mixture from the heat and allow to cool slightly – approximately 70 degrees.

- ➢ If you desire a specific color or fragrance for your soap you may add your favorite food coloring or essential oils to the mixture.

- ➢ Slowly pour the lye solution into the oil mixture.

- ➢ Stir until well blended

If the soap mixture does not thicken as desired within 30 minutes or there is a greasy layer on the top of the mixture it may be too warm.

> Set the container to cool in a pan of cool water.

> Continue stirring making sure to stir the sides and bottom of the pan to ensure an even mix. .

> The mixture will become thicker taking on the consistency of thick syrup.

If the soap mixture is too lumpy your mixture may be too cold. If this occurs, reverse the above process.

> Sit the mixture in a pan of warm water stirring until the lumps dissolve.

> Depending on the consistency you may need to replace your warm water more than once until the mixture is heated to the correct temperature for effective blending.

Once you have obtained the desired texture you may add fragrance or color to suit your desires.

Pour the thickened mixture into your molds and cover.

Keep the mixture in a warm place for at least 2 days.

This helps keep the mixture from separating.

The soaps on the following pages are variations on the basic soap recipes.

You can create your own soap, purchase melt and pour soap from a natural product supplier, or buy mass market soap that you will customize to suit your needs.

The variations on these pages are some of my favorite soap customizations. The ingredient mixes will work well with any of the core soap products described earlier.

Remember these are simply customizations I have created for my family and you can use the same process of replacement to customize the recipes to suit your needs.

Castile Soap

One of my favorite soaps is castile soap. To be considered castile soap the mixture must contain at least 40% olive oil. You can purchase ready made castile soap and then customize the mixture to suit your needs or you may create castile soap at home. Castile soap can be created in either liquid or solid cake form.

This soap is especially mild and gently and is excellent for children's soap mixtures. Castile soap is a versatile soap, you can even use the same castile soap products to wash your hair as you use for the rest of your body.

To create the solid form of castile soap the process is very similar to that of the other cake soap recipes included. The following recipe will yield approximately 1 bar of soap and can be enlarged to suit your desired quantity.

> Heat 1/3 cup olive oil to approximately 80 degrees Fahrenheit.

> While the oil is heating, dissolve 2 tsp. lye granules in 1/3 cup cold water.

> Remember to wear protective gloves and clothing when working with lye as lye can burn your skin. Store your unused lye granules in a safe place, as lye is a poison.

> Remove your oil mixture from the heat and allow to cool slightly – approximately 70 degrees.

> If you desire a specific color or fragrance for your soap you may add your favorite food coloring or essential oils to the mixture.

> Slowly pour the lye solution into the oil mixture.

> Stir the mixture gently but mix well to ensure all ingredients are well blended.

Soothing Oatmeal Soap

Perhaps my favorite modifications is a soothing oatmeal soap. Oatmeal is gentle, soothing and cleansing all at the same time. Oatmeal adds an exfoliating rub to the soap mixture while providing a soft, moist feel to my skin. Liquid based oatmeal soap is very versatile so a castile base is an excellent choice. I also love adding these ingredients to my coconut oil soap.

- ➢ 1 tsp.   Borax Powder

- ➢ 1/3 cup   Oil – Jojoba or Sesame Oil wok well

- ➢ 1 tsp.   Coconut Oil

Dissolve the borax powder in the oil base.

Borax in not a needed ingredient for this recipe but it can improve the appearance and performance of your soap.

Heat borax and oil mixture to approximately 80 degrees in your soap-making pan

Mix well and add

- ➢ 3 tsp.   Glycerin

- ➢ ¼ cup   Oatmeal

- ➢   Fragrance, Color, Emulsifier & Thickener as desired

Mix and pour into your favorite soap base.

You may need to heat the mixture a second time before blending with your soap base.

Continue stirring the mixture until well blended.

The mixture will become thicker taking on the consistency of thick syrup.

Moisturizing Age Reversing Bar

My mom loves this soap. It combines anti-aging properties with fantastic moisturizing components to make a nice daily soap that leaves her skin looking and feeling renewed.

The following recipe will yield approximately 1 bar of soap and can be enlarged to suit your desired quantity. I like to add these ingredients to my coconut or beeswax soap bars.

- ➢ 1/3 cup   Olive Oil

- ➢ 2 tsp.   Sea Buckthorn Oil

- ➢ 1 tsp.   Glycerin

Heat oils and glycerin to approximately 80 degrees Fahrenheit

- ➢ 3 tbsp.   Powdered Seaweed

- ➢ Fragrance, Color, Emulsifier & Thickener as desired

Dissolve seaweed into oil mixture making sure to distribute the powders evenly.

If you desire a specific color or fragrance for your soap you may add your favorite food coloring or essential oils to the mixture.

Slowly pour the soap solution of your choice into the oil mixture.

Mix well

Pour into molds and allow soap to harden

Pippen

Blushing Bride Soap

This is a great soap that I created for my sister to use the year she got married. It provides a well nourished glow to your skin. She looked fabulous and now uses the soap each day to provide a pretty, natural glow to her skin.

> 1/8 cup   Wheat Germ Oil

> 1/8 cup   Coconut Oil.

Heat the oils to approximately 80 degrees in your soap-making pan.

Add

> 1 tsp.   Carrot Juice

> 3 tbsp.   Watermelon Juice

> Fragrance, Color, Emulsifier & Thickener as desired

Stir juices into the oil mixture until well blended.

If you desire a specific color or fragrance for your soap you may add your favorite food coloring or essential oils to the mixture.

Pour the soap solution of your choice into the oil mixture.

Mix well

Pour into molds and allow soap to harden

Winter Wonder Soap

For skin that needs a little extra moisture this is a perfect soap. I use it during the winter months to provide extra moisturizing cleansing to my skin. I often use this soap for the babies in the family when their skin develops a rash or they are just cranky or irritable.

The following recipe will yield approximately one bar of soap and can be enlarged to suit your desired quantity.

- ➤ 3 tbsp.   Jojoba oil

- ➤ 3 tbsp.   Coconut Oil

- ➤ 2 tsp.   Lavender Oil

- ➤ ¼ cup   Lanolin Oil

Heat the oils over a low heat, stirring occasionally until they are approximately 75 degrees Fahrenheit.

- ➤ 2 tbsp.   Aloe Vera Gel

- ➤ Fragrance, Color, Emulsifier & Thickener as desired

Add aloe vera gel to mixture stirring until well blended.

If you desire a specific color or fragrance for your soap you may add your favorite food coloring or essential oils to the mixture.

Pour the soap solution of your choice into the oil mixture.

Mix well

Pour into molds and allow soap to harden

Wake-up Bars

My husband loves this soap. He is a slow starter in the morning. This soap is an invigorating body wash that wakes him up – plus it tightens the skin and minimizes the appearance of pores.

You can purchase ready made castile soap and then customize the mixture to suit your needs or you may create castile soap at home. We like to create this recipe in liquid from and apply with a scrubbing sack for the best benefits.

Create Castile Soap according to the recipe included earlier or buy pre-made castile soap from your favorite source.

> ➢ Add 2 tsp.   Menthol Oil to cooling mixture.

> ➢ Add 1 tsp   Mint Extract

> ➢ Fragrance, Color, Emulsifier & Thickener as desired

Stir well to ensure an even distribution.

Oil Reducing Soap

During the summer months when I am using a lot of extra moisturizer to counteract the damage our outdoor lifestyle does to my skin I often create an added problem of clogged pores and blemished skin.

➢ Heat 1/3 cup wheat germ oil to approximately 80 degrees in your soap-making pan.

➢ Remove your oil mixture from the heat and allow to cool slightly – approximately 70 degrees.

➢ Dissolve baking soda in oil mixture and add rosewater and pineapple juice to the solution.

3 tbsp.	Rosewater
3 tbsp.	Pineapple Juice
2 tbsp	Apricot Kernal Oil
2 tbsp.	Baking Soda

Fragrance, Color, Emulsifier & Thickener as desired

➢ If you desire a specific color or fragrance for your soap you may add your favorite food coloring or essential oils to the mixture.

➢ Pour the soap solution of your choice into the oil mixture.

➢ Mix well

➢ Pour into molds and allow soap to harden

Super Skin Clearing Bars

This soap works especially well for those with oily skin. I created this basic recipe for the teenagers in our family because it works very well in removing excess oils and clearing up minor skin blemishes.

- ➢ 1 tsp.   Borax Powder

- ➢ 2 tsp.   Sea Salt

- ➢ 3 tbsp.   Pineapple Juice

- ➢ 1 tbsp.   Honey

- ➢ Fragrance, Color, Emulsifier & Thickener as desired

Stir the Borax, Sea Salt, Pineapple Juice and honey into the soap base mixture until all ingredients are well blended.

If you desire a specific color or fragrance for your soap you may add your favorite food coloring or essential oils to the mixture.

Mix well

Pour into molds and allow soap to harden

Clarifying Bars

I like to use this soap once a week year round to clarify and tighten my skin. It also adds a lovely glowing look.

- ➢ 1/4 cup   Sesame Seed Oil

- ➢ 2 tbsp.   Grated Beeswax

- ➢ 1 tbsp.   Honey

Heat the mixture to approximately 90 degrees.

Remove your oil mixture from the heat and allow to cool slightly – approximately 70 degrees.   Add

- ➢ 2 tbsp.   Orange Flower Water

- ➢ 2 tsp.   Baking Soda

- ➢ 1 tsp.   Aluminum Sulfate

- ➢ 1 tsp.   Borax Powder

- ➢ 2 tsp.   Pineapple Juice

Use only USP Grade for Cosmetic use Aluminum Sulfate products. Mix ingredients in a plastic or ceramic dish with plastic utensils to avoid a reaction with metal.

If you desire a specific color or fragrance for your soap you may add your favorite food coloring or essential oils to the mixture.

Pour the soap solution of your choice into the oil mixture.

Mix well

Pour into molds and allow soap to harden

Anti-Bacterial Bath Bars

We wash our hands a lot during cold and flu season. I developed this recipe as an alternative to some of the harsher anti-bacterial soaps on the market and to obtain a gentle cleansing that provided additional protection to our skin.

> 1/4 cup   Almond Oil

> ¼ cup   Lanolin

> 4 tsp.   Grated Beeswax

Place oils and beeswax in your soap making pan and heat the mixture to approximately 90 degrees.

Remove your oil mixture from the heat and allow to cool slightly – approximately 70 degrees.

> 2 tbsp.   Honey

> 2 tbsp.   Glycerin

> 3 tbsp.   Lemon Juice

> Fragrance, Color, Emulsifier & Thickener as desired

Add the honey, glycerin and lemon juice to the oil and beeswax mixture stirring until well blended.

If you desire a specific color or fragrance for your soap you may add your favorite food coloring or essential oils to the mixture.

Pour the soap solution of your choice into the oil mixture.

Mix well

Pour into molds and allow soap to harden

Muscle Balm Soap

We have a very active lifestyle and there are some mornings when my muscles ache and I just don't want to wake up. Anytime I am tired and sore this particular soap becomes a favorite. It provides a soothing muscle was while the scent invigorates and provides a more alert frame of mind. I prefer this as a liquid soap so that I can massage it into my aching muscles while showering.

- ➢ 3 tsp.   Lavender Oil

- ➢ 3 tsp.   Coconut Oil

- ➢ ¼ cup   Vegetable Based Shortening

Heat the oils and shortening over a low heat, stirring occasionally until approximately 75 degrees Fahrenheit.

Remove your oil mixture from the heat and allow to cool slightly – approximately 70 degrees.

- ➢ 1 ½ tsp.   Eucalyptus Oil

- ➢ 1 ½ tsp.   Menthol Crystals

- ➢ Fragrance, Color, Emulsifier & Thickener as desired

Stir the eucalyptus oil and menthol crystals into your heated oil mixture until well blended. Do not add these oils before heating because much of the medicinal qualities can be lost during the heating process.

Pour the soap solution of your choice into the oil mixture.

Mix well

Pour into molds and allow soap to harden

Bedtime Bars

This is a favorite of mine at night before bed. The natural aroma of chamomile is believed to provide a relaxing benefit while the soap itself softens and hydrates my skin. I typically follow this treatment with a hydrating moisturizer and wake with beautiful, moisturized skin.

- ➢ 1 tbsp.   Chamomile Leaves (1 teabag)

- ➢ 1/8 cup   Water

Heat water to the boiling point and pour over the chamomile leaves. Allow the leaves and water to soak overnight. The mixture should form a tea.

- ➢ 1 tbsp.   Coconut Oil

- ➢ 1/3 cup   Jojoba Oil

- ➢ 1 tbsp.   Wheat Germ Oil

- ➢ 1 tsp.   Borax Powder

Dissolve the borax powder in the oil base. Borax in not a needed ingredient for this recipe but it can improve the appearance and performance of your soap. Heat borax and oil mixture to approximately 80 degrees in your soap-making pan

Remove mixture from heat and allow to cool slightly – approximately 70 degrees.

- ➢ 1/8 cup   Carrot Juice

Add carrot juice to cooling oils stirring until well blended.

If you desire a specific color or fragrance for your soap you may add your favorite food coloring or essential oils to the mixture.

When the ingredients are well blended add the remaining ingredients and mix well.

- ➢ 3 tsp.   Glycerin.

- ➢ ¼ cup   Oatmeal

- ➢ Fragrance, Color, Emulsifier & Thickener as desired

Pour the soap solution of your choice into the oil mixture.

Mix well

Pour into molds and allow soap to harden

Summer Balm Soap

Both summer and winter whenever my skin is chapped and sore or even sunburned this is the soap of choice. I also use this whenever our children have a rash that needs soothed.

- ¼ cup   Jojoba Oil

- ¼ cup   Wheat Germ Oil

- ¼ cup   Aloe Vera gel

- Fragrance, Color, Emulsifier & Thickener as desired

Heat the oil and aloe mixture to approximately 80 degrees in your soap-making pan.

Remove your oil mixture from the heat and allow to cool slightly – approximately 70 degrees.

If you desire a specific color or fragrance for your soap you may add your favorite food coloring or essential oils to the mixture.

Pour the soap solution of your choice into the oil mixture.

Mix well

Pour into molds and allow soap to harden

Apple Soap

Another excellent choice for irritated skin is apple juice based soap. This is great when you have an itchy rash, especially diaper rash.

- ➢ 1/3 cup   Lanolin

- ➢ 4 tsp.   Grated Beeswax

Heat lanolin and beeswax until melted to a loose liquid; the mixture will be approximately 90 degrees.

Remove your oil mixture from the heat and allow to cool slightly – approximately 70 degrees.

- ➢ 2 tbsp.   Apple Juice

- ➢ 1 tsp.   Liquid Chlorophyll

- ➢ Fragrance, Color, Emulsifier & Thickener as desired

Add apple juice and chlorophyll to your lanolin and beeswax mixture, stirring until well blended.

The mixture will have a delicate apple scent and a lovely green color. If you desire a different color or fragrance you may add food coloring or the desired essential oils to the mixture.

Pour the soap solution of your choice into the oil mixture.

Mix well

Pour into molds and allow soap to harden

Hydrating Bars

This soap is great to hydrate and exfoliate all in one plus provides a gentle clean feeling to the skin. You will be amazed at how moist and clear you skin looks after using this soap.

- ➢ 1 tsp.   Borax Powder

- ➢ 1/3 cup   Sesame Seed Oil

- ➢ 1 tsp.   Coconut Oil

- ➢ 2 tsp.   Grated Beeswax

Dissolve the borax powder in the oil base. Borax in not a needed ingredient for this recipe but it can improve the appearance and performance of your soap. Heat borax and oil mixture to approximately 80 degrees in your soap-making pan

- ➢ 2 tsp.   Lye Granules

- ➢ 1/3 cup   Cold Water

Remove your oil mixture from the heat and allow to cool slightly – approximately 70 degrees.

- ➢ 1/8 cup   Carrot Juice

Add carrot juice to your oil solution. Stir until well blended.

The mixture will have an orange appearance. If you desire a specific color or fragrance for your soap you may add your favorite food coloring or essential oils to the mixture.

Pour the soap solution of your choice into the oil mixture.

Mix well

When the ingredients are well blended, add the remaining ingredients and mix well.

> 3 tsp. glycerin.

> 1 orange peel grated medium fine

> Fragrance, Color, Emulsifier & Thickener as desired

Continue stirring the mixture until well blended. The mixture will become thicker taking on the consistency of thick syrup.

Pour into molds and allow to cool.

Soothing Bath Balm

While any soap may be turned into a liquid by dissolving the hardened cakes in water there is one particular liquid soap I prefer. Almost anytime I have a recipe that lends itself to liquid form I use this recipe as a base. Alone this is a gentle, moisturizing cleanser that soothes and protects your skin.

- ¼ cup   Aloe Vera Gel

- 1 tbsp.   Vitamin E Oil

- 2 tbsp.   Borax Powder

- 2 tbsp.   Powdered Milk

- ¼ cup   Witch Hazel

- Fragrance, Color, Emulsifier & Thickener as desired

Dissolve Borax Powder and milk powder in the witch hazel base. Add remaining ingredients and blend well.

If you desire a specific color or fragrance for your soap you may add your favorite food coloring or essential oils to the mixture.

Pour into clean container and seal tightly. To use pour small amount in the palm of your hand or apply to your favorite scrubbing sacks

CHAPTER 8

Bath Treatments

The appearance of skin is as important as the health of your skin. There are many steps and processes involved in the proper care of skin. Each person will have different needs they desire from their skin care regimen.

Skin care products are perhaps the most customizable of all of the products included in this book. Some people will require anti-acne treatments, while others may need a product that hydrates. One person may desire anti-aging treatments while another person's prime focus may be on cellulite reducing products.

Each chapter in this book relates to the appearance and health of your skin. This next chapter will provide you with general body care products that can be used daily.

Each treatment will provide a different effect and a different benefit. The primary key to beautiful skin is to keep it clean and full of moisture.

There are products that clean, nourish, exfoliate and moisturize the skin.

Bath time is one of my favorite times to pamper my skin. I love combining the peaceful relaxation of a bath with the beneficial effects of my favorite products.

Skin Soothing Soak

This is an excellent bath additive I like to use when my skin is irritated from sunburns or other environmental factors or just to relax. This is also an excellent recipe to add to the baby bath to help soothe a cranky baby or help relieve skin issues such as diaper rash.

- ➤ 4 tbsp.   Lavender Oil

- ➤ ¼ cup   Apple Juice

- ➤ ¼ cup   Witch Hazel

- ➤ ¼ cup   Aloe Vera Gel

- ➤ ¼ cup   Epsom Salts

Dissolve salts in witch hazel base.

Add the remaining ingredients and mix until well blended.

Pour into a clean container and seal tightly.

Part of the benefit of this treatment comes from the scent released from the lavender oils. If you desire the skin benefits without the sedative and relaxing qualities of the lavender aroma you may exchange the lavender with your favorite scent.

Food coloring may also be added at this time to create a pretty color to your recipe and the bathwater.

Shake well before using.

Add approximately ¼ cup to warm bathwater and soak 10-15 minutes until desired soothing effect has been achieved.

Fountain of Youth Bath

This is a wonderful bath additive for people of all ages. The chamomile and carrot juice aid in skin hydration while the oils gently bath your skin in moisture. The combination of seaweed and alum powder helps tighten and tone her skin giving it a hydrated and youthful glow.

- ➤ 1 tbsp.   Dried Chamomile (1 teabag)

- ➤ ¼ cup   Boiling Water

Pour water over chamomile leaves and allow to soak overnight.

A strong tea should be created.

Strain leaves from water and discard.

- ➤ ¼ cup   Carrot

- ➤ 1/8 cup   Seaweed Powder

- ➤ ½ cup   Wheat Germ Oil

- ➤ 1 tsp.   Alum Powder

Use only USP Grade for Cosmetic Use Alum Powder.

Add remaining ingredients to the tea solution and mix until well blended.

The mixture will have the soothing scent of chamomile but if you desire a specific color or fragrance you may add your favorite food coloring or essential oils to the mixture.

Pour finished mixture into a clean container and seal tightly.

To use pour approximately ¼ cup into warm bath and soak approximately 10-15 minutes.

Simple Hydrating Bath

I love this bath to hydrate my skin whenever I have been doing a lot of outdoor activities. Hydrated skin looks healthier and more youthful and gains back its ability to retain moisture.

> 2 tbsp.   Chamomile Leaves (2 teabags)

> ½ cup   Boiling Water

Pour boiling water over chamomile and let steep overnight.

Strain the chamomile leaves and discard.

> ½ cup   Carrot Juice

Add carrot juice to the chamomile liquid and blend.

Your recipe will be orange in color and have a slight aroma; however you may alter the color or fragrance if desired by adding food coloring or your favorite essential oils.

Pour solution into your favorite container and seal tightly.

Shake well before using.

Pour ½ mixture into warm bath and soak 15-20 minutes. F

Follow with a deep moisturizer for best results.

Skin Clarifying Soak

Sometimes my skin becomes oversaturated with oils from sunscreen lotions or other products that I apply in an effort to improve the look and feel of my skin. I often use a clarifying product once or twice a month to counter any negative effects of some of the products I use. This is also an excellent solution for those with oily skin or body blemishes since it aids in removing surface dirt and oils and helps unclog pores.

- ¼ cup   Vinegar

- 1 cup   Orange Flower Water

- ½ cup   Rosewater

- ¼ cup   Sea Salts

Dissolve salts in liquid and shake solution until well blended.

The recipe will have a stronger vinegar smell so you may want to add your favorite fragrances to your solution to alter the smell.

Food coloring may also be added to provide a pretty color to your recipe and your bath water.

Pour into a clean container and seal tightly.

You will want to shake the solution before using to ensure the ingredients are well blended.

To use add approximately ¼ cup to your bath and soak approximately 15-20 minutes.

If your skin is not oily you should follow this treatment with a light moisturizer.

Youthful Milk Bath

Milk has long been believed to provide exceptional beauty benefits. This recipe combines the best of the milk and yogurt products with oils and humectants which will provide a lovely moist glow to your skin. I use this bath as often as I can to give my skin a beautiful smooth texture.

- ¼ cup   Plain Yogurt
- ¼ cup   Powdered Milk
- 1 tbsp   Wheat Germ Oil
- 1 tbsp.   Glycerin
- 1 tbsp.   Honey

Combine the ingredients stirring gently until well blended.

If you desire a specific color or fragrance you may add your favorite food coloring or essential oils to the mixture.

Pour into a tightly sealed container and store in the refrigerator until ready to use.

Add 5-6 tbsp to your bath for soaking.

I love to smooth the mixture over my skin with a scrubbing sack for added penetration.

Basic Bubble Bath

This is a great basic bubble bath that is suitable for both children and adults. There is nothing I find more relaxing than soaking in a tub full of bubbles.

> ➤ ¼ cup   Liquid Castile Soap

> ➤ 1 pack   Unflavored Gelatin

> ➤ 1 tbsp   Glycerin

> ➤ 1 tbsp.   Jojoba Oil

> ➤ 2 tbsp.   Coconut Oil

Combine the ingredients and gently mix until well blended. Do not whip the mixture as it will foam.

If you desire a specific color or fragrance you may add your favorite food coloring or essential oils to the mixture.

Pour into tightly sealed container and store.

To use pour mixture as desired under the running water used to fill your bath.

You may want to add your favorite essential oil our fragrance to the mixture for a customized bath.

Muscle Soothing Soak

This is a great bath soak for sore, tired muscles. I also love using this solution when I am sick with a cold or flu since the camphor provides a great aroma for clearing my head and chest and the recipe goes a long way toward soothing the aches and pain that result from many illnesses.

- ½ cup   Liquid Castile Soap

- 2 packs   Unflavored Gelatin

- 1 tbsp.   Glycerin

- 2 tbsp.   Camphor Oil

- ¼ cup   Epsom Salts

Dissolve salts and gelatin into castile soap.

Add glycerin and camphor.

Blend well

The finished product will have the smell of camphor which can provide medicinal benefits.

If you desire a specific color or fragrance you may add your favorite food coloring or essential oils to the mixture.

Pour into a clean container and seal tightly.

To use pour desired amount into the bath water as you fill your tub.

Soak 15-20 minutes until desired results have been achieved.

Soothing Salts

This is an excellent bath salt that I like to use anytime my skin needs a little pampering. It also works well as a scrub.

- ➢ 1 cup   Epsom Salts

- ➢ 1 cup   Uncooked Oatmeal

- ➢ 2 tsp.   Avocado Oil

Combine the dry ingredients in a container.

Pour oils over mixture and shake until the oils are evenly distributed.

You can add your favorite scent and color to the mixture to customize the salts to suit your needs.

To add a fragrance or color sprinkle the desired item over the mixture similar to the way you mixed the oils.

Shake well to evenly distribute the color or fragrance and seal the container tightly.

To use pour approximately ¼ cup in warm bath water for a soothing soak or rub a handful of the mixture over the skin for an excellent shower or bath scrub.

Relaxing Bath Crystals

These are an excellent bath additive that I use whenever I need extra relaxation. The components also provide a moisturizing hydration that leaves the skin feeling soft and looking great.

- ¾ cup   Epsom salts

- ¼ cup   Sea Salts

- 1 tsp.   Favorite Essential Oils

- 2 tbsp.   Dried Chamomile Flowers

Crush the chamomile flowers to a fine dust.

Place the salts and chamomile powder in a container, seal and shake until well blended.

Pour oils over the mixture. You can use any oil whose scent and benefits suit your needs.

Stir the oils into the salt mixture until they are evenly distributed.

I like to add a few drops of food color to my salts when I add the oils giving my salts and therefore my bath a pretty color.

Seal the container tightly and add a handful of crystals to your bath anytime you want a relaxing soak.

Colored and scented bath salts make excellent gifts for friends and family, especially when oils that match that person's preference are used.

I like to purchase pretty jars and bottles and give them as additions to every gift for special occasions.

Age Defying Bath Balm

This is a wonderful mixture that I like to use whenever I have a formal event to attend that requires my skin be tight and toned. It is also great before a pool party.

> - 2 cups   Sea Salt
>
> - 1 tbsp.   Powdered Seaweed
>
> - ¼ cup   Rosewater
>
> - 4 tbsp.   Clary Sage
>
> - 2 tbsp   Sunflower Oil

Mix the dry ingredients until well blended.

Dissolve the salt and powder in the rosewater then add the oil until well blended.

The mixture will form a paste.

Spoon the mixture into a clean container and seal tightly.

If you desire a specific color or fragrance you may add your favorite food coloring or essential oils to the mixture.

To use add ¼ cup of the salt mixture to your bath or use a handful as a rub directly on your skin.

Do not rinse the solution after bathing.

Cellulite Reduction Bath Powder

This is an excellent powder to add to your bath if you have a special event or occasion and want smooth skin and to minimize the appearance of cellulite. The tightening action of the seaweed powder will help reduce the appearance of cellulite on skin and promotes a more youthful appearance.

> ¼ cup   Powdered Seaweed

> ½ cup   Cornstarch

Blend the dry ingredients until evenly distributed.

If you desire a specific color or fragrance for your soap you may add your favorite food coloring or essential oils to the mixture.

Sprinkle a few drops of your chosen color or fragrance over the mixture and shake or stir the mixture until the color or fragrance is evenly distributed.

Store in a clean, tightly sealed container

Add ¼ cup of the mixture to your bath and soak approximately 20-30 minutes.

Follow the bath with an age minimizing moisturizer for best results.

Ivy Bath Soak

English Ivy is an excellent product for use for special occasions. The ivy helps draw fluids from the skin and reduces the appearance of cellulite while providing a more youthful appearance to the skin.

- ➢ 10   English Ivy Leaves
- ➢ ½ cup   Boiling Water

Pour water over Ivy leaves and allow to soak for 24-36 hours. Strain the leaves from the water and discard.

- ➢ ¼ cup   Wheat Germ Oil
- ➢ 3 tbsp.   Seaweed Powder

Add the oil and powder to your ivy water and blend ingredients until well mixed.

If you desire a specific color or fragrance for your soap you may add your favorite food coloring or essential oils to the mixture.

Pour solution into clean container and seal tightly.

To use shake well and pour ¼ cup into your bath

Soak 20-30 minutes.

Follow with an age minimizing moisturizer for the best effect.

Nighttime Bath for Damaged Skin

This is an excellent balm for irritated or injured skin. I keep this mixed and available during the summer months to soak in the event of sunburn. We have also found this provides an excellent soothing bath if you have eczema or a rash caused by poison ivy or oak.

- ¼ cup Dried Marigold
- ½ cup Boiling Water

Pour water over marigolds and allow solution to steep 24-36 hours.

Strain the marigolds from the water and discard.

- 2 tbsp. Almond Oil
- 3 tbsp. Coconut Oil
- 1 tbsp. Glycerin
- 1 packet Unflavored Gelatin
- 3 tbsp. Aloe Vera Gel

Combine the remaining ingredients with the marigold water stirring until well blended.

The mixture will have a slight aroma from the almond oil and the marigolds. If you desire a specific color or fragrance you may add your favorite food coloring or essential oils to the mixture.

Pour into a container and seal tightly.

To use add ¼ cup of the liquid to your warm bath water and soak until relief is obtained.

You may need to repeat the process if the skin is especially irritated or sore.

Foaming Bath Gel

I love using this gel in my winter bath water, though it works equally well in the shower. The mixture has an excellent foaming effect while providing a moisturizing, protecting film to your skin.

- ➤ 4 tbsp.   Grated Beeswax

- ➤ 1 cup   Coconut Oil

Heat beeswax and oil in the microwave in a microwave safe dish until melted approximately 20 seconds on medium heat

- ➤ ½ tbsp   Gelatin Powder (approximately ½ packet)

- ➤ 3 tsp.   Borax Powder

- ➤ 2 tbsp.   Honey

Mix remaining ingredients with the heated oils until well blended.

If you desire a specific color or fragrance you may add your favorite food coloring or essential oils to the mixture.

Pour into a pump container and use as desired.

To use pump one or two squirts into the palm of your hand and apply directly to the skin.

The mixture will foam a great deal and should not be fully rinsed from the skin as the film left from the oils will provide a moisturizing, protective film.

Hydrating Bath Oil

Skin hydration is essential to a nice appearance. This is a great additive for every bath.

- ¼ cup   Dried Chamomile Leaves
- ½ cup   Boiling Water

Pour water over chamomile leaves and allow mixture to steep overnight. Strain the leaves from the water and discard.

- ½ cup   Safflower Oil
- ¼ cup   Avocado Oil
- ¼ cup   Carrot Juice

Combine remaining ingredients with the chamomile tea mixture and stir until well blended.

The mixture will have an orange color and a delicate scent. If you desire a different fragrance or color you may add your favorite essential oil or food coloring to achieve the desired effect.

Pour into clean container and seal tightly.

To use shake well and add ¼ cup of the liquid to your bath

Soak 10-15 minutes.

Do not rinse solution from the skin.

Uplifting Memory Bath

This is an excellent additive to your bath that can also be used as soap for your shower. I love to use this anytime I need a pick me up especially when memory enhancement is desired. The herbs included are believed to lift your spirits while stimulating your mind and invigorating your body. I actually call this mixture my "meeting soap" around the house since I use it anytime I have an important meeting or presentation.

- ¼ cup   Ground Mint Leaves

- ¼ cup   Ground Rosemary

- 4 tbsp.   Basil

- 4 tbsp.   Ground Sage

As a bath additive the herbs can be combined and tossed into a warm bath for a lovely aromatic and effective aroma. You might also blend the herbs and put them in a scrubbing sack. I like to use mine in the morning in place of my normal soap so I modify the recipe even further.

- 1 cup Castile Soap

- ½ cup   Warm Water

Pour the blended herbs into the castile soap and water mixture.

Blend well.

One of the primary benefits of this recipe is derived from the combination of scents from the herbs. Alterations to the fragrance are not recommended.

You may add your favorite color to the mixture by adding a few drops of food coloring and mixing well.

Pour into a clean container. Seal tightly.

To use shake well and pour a small amount into the palm of your hand

CHAPTER 9

Body Wraps & Treatment

At times specific areas of the skin will require specialized treatments. Women pay hundreds of dollars at spas every day to obtain only one of the treatments in this chapter. There are many treatments included but be sure to experiment with the alternate ingredient list to custom create your own personalized spa experience.

For specific, health related concerns; you should always consult your physician to determine the best course of action for you. For cosmetic and more minor concerns many of the recipes included in this chapter provide exceptional benefits. These recipes are also an excellent way to pamper yourself and just relax! For special holidays when my husband asks what I want for a gift I always ask for a day at home alone so I can experiment with new treatments and spend all the time I want using treatments I know I love. This is the best gift I ever got!

Cellulite Reduction Wrap

This body wrap is a fantastic discovery that actually helps reduce the appearance of cellulite. English Ivy helps remove retained water from the skin and minimize the look of cellulite. I love to use a wrap like this as often as I can in the summer because summer wear can show off every flaw or it can show off beautiful toned skin!

- ½ cup   Powdered Clay

- ¼ cup   Carrot Juice

- ¼ cup   Warm Water

- 10   Finely Ground English Ivy Leaves

- 1 tbsp.   Wheat Germ Oil

- 2 tbsp.   Sea Salt

Mix the carrot juice and the water with the wheat germ oil.

Dissolve the sea salt in the liquid solution and then add the English Ivy Powder.

Slowly add the clay powder until a thick paste is formed.

The product will have its own natural scent and color, but if you desire a specific color to suit your needs or an aromatherapy benefit you may add your favorite colorant or essential oils to the recipe.

Apply in an even coat all over your skin.

Wrap yourself in a warm towel or saran wrap as desired.

Allow the mixture to soak into your skin for approximately 30 minutes or until the clay begins to dry.

Rinse clay from skin and pat dry.

Skin Renewal Body Mask

This is another exceptional body mask that is very popular in day spas. The mask extracts toxins from below the surface of the skin and providing a beautiful clear glow while softening the surface of the skin and infusing it with moisture. I love to use this one at least once a month to keep my skin clear and glowing.

- ½ cup — Powdered Clay
- ¼ cup — Powdered Kelp (seaweed)
- 2 tbsp. — Sea Salt
- ¼ cup — Water
- 3 tbsp. — Sesame Seed Oil
- ¼ cup — Aloe Vera Gel

Blend the water, aloe vera gel and oil with the sea salt and powdered kelp.

Stir until the powder and salts are dissolved.

Slowly add the clay powder until a thick paste is formed and all ingredients are moist and well mixed.

If the powder is too dry and flaky add small amounts of water until the correct texture is achieved.

The product will have its own natural scent and color, but if you desire a specific color to suit your needs or an aromatherapy benefit you may add your favorite colorant or essential oils to the recipe.

Spread the clay mixture all over your body. I like to use a sea sponge to spread the mixture but you may use any applicator that is available.

Allow the mask to dry and harden – approximately 15-20 minutes. Rinse and pat the skin dry. I typically follow this treatment with a moisture rich lotion since this mixture tends to leave my skin type a little dry.

Exfoliation is the process of removing dead cells and impurities from the surface of the skin. This is a very important process to obtaining the healthy, glowing skin you desire. Exfoliation not only removes dead cells and impurities, but the process of removing these cells actually allows your skin to retain moisture and for the appearance of brand new cells. These specialized products may be used in place of or in addition to your regular daily soap. Many of the products included in this chapter are designed for the bath but can be used as a shower treatment as well.

Body Scrubs

I love to have a handful of grains available to scrub my face and body each day. I use these scrubs before my soap to remove any surface dirt and oils and to gently exfoliate my skin in preparation for the remaining treatments in my daily regimen.

There are a variety of cleansing grains you can use but the easiest to find and the ones I have found the most effective are:

> ➤ Uncooked Oatmeal

> ➤ Cornmeal

> ➤ Wheat Germ

You may combine these grains or use them individually for great results. To use combine the grains with warm water to create a paste. Massage the mixture into your skin in a gentle rub. Rinse well and follow with your favorite daily treatments.

Sometimes the loose grains are messy so I use a bag to apply the grains. To make a scrubbing bag take any material you desire, I prefer using old panty hose cut to size but gauze or cheesecloth squares work well. Mix your favorite grains, grated soaps and oils together in a bowl and spoon the mixture onto your chosen cloth. Tie the cloth closed and you have an excellent rubbing bag for your bath.

The product will have its own natural scent and color, but if you desire a specific color to suit your needs or an aromatherapy benefit you may add your favorite colorant or essential oils to the recipe.

Rough Skin Grain Bag

I have a particular grain mixture that I like to use in my scrubbing sacks. The grains work well all by themselves, but I have customized the ingredients to provide some additional benefits. This is a fantastic cleansing scrub that provides a lovely moisturized texture to my skin. The grains gently exfoliate and the oils infuse the newly bared skin with moisture. I use this combination on the rougher areas of my skin such as the elbows and the feet. These areas often need special attention and this allows me to combine the treatment steps during the busy work week when I might otherwise skip the vital steps that help keep these areas soft and pretty.

- ¼ tsp. Borax Powder

- ¼ cup   Wheat Germ Oil

- 1 tsp.   Ground Sage

- ¼ cup   Oatmeal

- ¼ cup   Cornmeal

- 1 tsp.   Honey

Blend the dry ingredients until they are well mixed. Slowly pour the oils and honey over the dry ingredients and mix to distribute the oils evenly.

Place 3-4 tbsp. of the mixture on your favorite bag making cloth and tie the cloth closed. I like to attach a string to make the cloth easier to hang.

The product will have its own natural scent and color, but if you desire a specific color to suit your needs or an aromatherapy benefit you may add your favorite colorant or essential oils to the recipe.

To use moisten the cloth and massage into the desired areas. I use this bag specifically on the rough, dry patches of my skin but it works well all over the body and face. Dry the bag between uses to ensure the longest shelf life possible.

Exfoliation Rub

Fruit pits contain many of the same benefits and oils as the fruit itself or even the oil extracted from the fruit. I like to have a stronger exfoliation scrub available for more focused care of the rougher patches of my skin such as elbows, knees and feet.

There are a variety of fruit pits you will see available in the scrubs sold at your local stores.

Avocado Pit: Very rich in oils that provide exceptional skin softening and conditioning with a more abrasive rub

Apricot Kernel: Perhaps the easiest oils for the skin to absorb, these are rich in Vitamin A which is vital for healthy, glowing skin

Peach Pit: Rich in conditioning oils that will aid in keeping skin soft and supple while acting as mild humectants to attract additional oils to the surface of the skin.

To create a scrub, remove the hard shell from the outside of the pit or seed.

Inside the hard shell will be an oil rich nut like product.

Grind the nut to the desired consistency.

 The larger the finished pieces the courser your abrasive action will be.

For normal skin grind the pits to a loose powder similar in texture to corn meal.

The product will have its own natural scent and color, but if you desire a specific color to suit your needs or an aromatherapy benefit you may add your favorite colorant or essential oils to the recipe.

You can use the scrubs alone or mix them with a cold cream or soap for a foaming action. You may also place your ground pits in a scrubbing bag for easier and cleaner application. Just be sure your chosen bag has large enough mesh to allow the pits abrasive action to come through.

Rough Foot Intensive Treatment

This is a great cleansing scrub that will gently remove surface dirt and dried skin cells. I like this treatment because it is very soothing to the rough skin of my feet. You can apply this mix to any area of your body that needs extra work. If you are applying this to your face or more sensitive skin be sure to grind the finished product to a finer consistency. The larger the pieces the harsher the abrasive action.

- 3 tbsp.   Almond Oil

- 2 tbsp.   Ground Almond (almond meal may be used if desired)

- ¼ cup   Aloe Vera Gel

- 3 tbsp.   Witch Hazel Gel

Mix all ingredients until well blended.

The product will have its own natural scent and color, but if you desire a specific color to suit your needs or an aromatherapy benefit you may add your favorite colorant or essential oils to the recipe.

Pour into a clean container and seal tightly.

To use massage mixture into the desired area

The mixture will seem a bit rough because of the ground almonds but remember it is that abrasive action that provides the exfoliating action.

If the mixture is courser than desired you may place all of the ingredients in the blender and gently blend until the desired consistency is reached.

Mermaid Bath Rub

Mermaids are said to have beautiful, glowing skin. Perhaps this is a result of the salt water that they call home. This is another treatment that is very popular in the spas of the United States and Europe. The rub gently removes skin surface dirt and dead skin cells and then laves the newly revealed skin in easily absorbed oils. This treatment can be irritating to irritated or damaged skin so only use this if your skin is already in good condition.

- ½ cup   Sea Salt

- ½ cup   Epsom Salts

- ½ cup   Apricot Kernel Oil

- 1 tsp.   Vitamin E Oil

Mix the salts and oils until they are well blended and form a thick paste.

The product will have its own natural scent and color, but if you desire a specific color to suit your needs or an aromatherapy benefit you may add your favorite colorant or essential oils to the recipe.

Spoon the paste into a clean container and seal tightly.

To use massage a handful of the paste into your skin.

Start at the top of your body and work your way to your feet.

The oils will make your skin and tub very slippery.

Massage the paste into your body.

When you reach your feet, rinse your skin well and pat dry.

Do not use soap following this treatment because it will minimize the effects.

Citrus Scrub

This is a great scrub that has a pretty clean scent and provides moisture to dry, rough skin while gently removing dead cells to reveal fresher, younger looking skin. I like to use this in combination with some of my other citrus based products to provide an all over body theme to the day. The peels are rich in oils and anti-oxidants and the lemon and pineapple juice provides a clarifying bath.

- ➢ 1 tsp.   Lemon Juice

- ➢ ¼ tsp. Borax Powder

- ➢ ¼ cup   Pineapple Juice

- ➢ ¼ cup   Mineral Oil

- ➢ ¼ cup   Aloe Vera Gel

Blend the ingredients until they are well mixed.

- ➢ orange or lemon peel – colored and white portion – finely ground

Mix the orange peel into the cream mixture.

The product will have its own natural scent and color, but if you desire a specific color to suit your needs or an aromatherapy benefit you may add your favorite colorant or essential oils to the recipe.

Stir the ground peel into the mixture and pour into a clean container. Seal tightly.

To apply, shake mixture well and massage a handful into your skin.

Rinse and pat skin dry

I like to follow this treatment with a citrus scented lotion for extra conditioning.

Foot Refresher

This rub is fantastic when my feet and legs ache. I often spend the whole day on the move on my feet. By the end of the day there are few things I want more than to put my feet up and relax. This is one of those few things. Massage this rub into your feet and legs. You will be amazed at how refreshed and invigorated this makes those tired, aching feet!

- ➢ 1 tsp.   Borax Powder

- ➢ ¼ cup   Witch Hazel

- ➢ 3 tbsp.   Cucumber Juice

- ➢ ¼ cup   Aloe Vera Gel

- ➢ 1 tsp.   Stearic Acid

- ➢ ¼ cup   Epsom Salts

Combine all ingredients, stirring until well blended.

You may add your favorite color or fragrance to improve the effect.

I like to use a mint oil to add an invigorating aroma to go with the invigorating feeling.

Pour into a clean container and seal tightly.

To use gently massage a small amount into your feet and legs and relax.

Do not rinse since the solutions effect on the skin and muscles will continue beyond the massage.

I like to follow this with an invigorating moisturizer.

Summer Refreshing Gel

Sometimes my skin and body need a refreshing healing rub. I sometimes use one designed for my feet and leg all over my body but this one works wonders too. The cornstarch makes my skin feel super soft and the other ingredients help heal damage caused by the sun and provide a clean refreshing feeling at the same time.

- ➢ ½ cup   Aloe Vera Gel

- ➢ 3 tsp.   Cornstarch

- ➢ 1 tbsp.   Witch Hazel

Combine the ingredients in a microwave safe dish.

Heat on medium approximately 45 seconds until mixture is a syrupy liquid.

Remove from microwave and allow the mixture to cool.

- ➢ ½ tsp.   Spearmint oils or Eucalyptus Oil
  (you may use another invigorating essential oil)

Stir oils into cooled mixture and pour into a clean container.

Seal tightly.

Massage this mixture into your arms, legs and feet for a cooling refresher any time or into damaged skin for a refreshing balm that provides relief for sun damaged skin.

Stretch Mark Cream

Every woman knows that stretch marks are often a side effect of pregnancy. I used this cream as often as possible when I was pregnant to help minimize the appearance and even to avoid getting them in the first place. Dieters are often surprised to find they get stretch marks when they lose weight. Stretch marks cannot be removed once they have appeared, but they can fade over time. The best plan is to avoid their appearance in the first place. This is an oily cream but the oily feel is definitely worth avoiding the appearance of stretch marks.

> ¼ cup   Cocoa Butter

> 1 tsp.   Vitamin E Oil

> 1 tsp.   Apricot Kernel Oil

> 1 tbsp.   Wheat Germ Oil

> 1 tbsp.   Jojoba Oil

> 1 tsp.   Aloe Vera Gel

> 1 tbsp.   Grated Beeswax

> 1 tsp.   Glycerin

Measure all ingredients into a microwave safe dish.

Heat the mixture until the cocoa butter and beeswax are melted to a thick syrup.

Stir all ingredients until well blended.

The product will have its own natural scent and color, but if you desire a specific color to suit your needs or an aromatherapy benefit you may add your favorite colorant or essential oils to the recipe. Pour into a clean container and allow the mixture to cool. This will be a firmer mixture.

Massage the lotion into the effected skin areas as frequently as possible during periods when stretch mark appearance is likely.

Antibacterial Wash, Cream, and Soap

Anti bacterial hand washes and creams are becoming very popular. Because this is a simple product to create at home and is much used in today's households, we are devoting a section just toward wash, lotion and soaps that contain anti-bacterial properties.

Many of the products on the market today are alcohol based. This means that they can be irritating to dry or sensitive skin or have a strong smell that some people find unpleasant. There are many natural products that have antibacterial properties. You can use these products to create your own personalized line of anti-bacterial washes, soaps and lotions.

We have included some basic recipes to get you started. You will want to review the ingredients listing for this section very carefully to determine which other natural anti-bacterial products might work best for you and which might not work for you and your family. Most of the ingredients included in the listing can be added to your favorite recipes from other sections of the book to create your very own anti bacterial personal care line.

Waterless Hand Lotion

Anti-aging and moisturizing with anti-bacterial properties

Many of the waterless hand lotions on the market are very drying to my skin. Dry and aged looking hands are a problem in my family so I am always experimenting with products that provide the benefits I need without undue drying and aging to my hands. This works well, providing both anti-aging components with moisturizing and anti-bacterial properties

> ➢ 2 tbsp   Grated Beeswax

> ➢ 2 tbsp   Liquid or Grated Lecithin

Combine beeswax and lecithin in a microwave safe dish and microwave on medium approximately 20 seconds until mixture is creamy.

> ➢ ¼ tsp   Aluminum Sulfate Powder

> ➢ 3 tbsp   Aloe Vera Gel

> ➢ 1 tsp   Orange Flower Water

Blend all ingredients in a bowl. Stirring gently until well mixed.

Pour the mixture into your favorite container or pump and use as desired.

Pump or pour about a dime size portion into the palm of your hand and rub until skin is well coated.

Lavender Moisturizing Antibacterial Waterless Wash

This is a nice waterless wash I like to use for the soothing effects of Lavender. I also use it as a bath additive when the kids are especially fussy or ill and need a relaxing bath to help prepare them for bed.

- ¼ tsp — Tincture of Benzoin
- 1 tbsp — Distilled Water
- 3 tbsp — Witch Hazel
- 3-4 drops — Lavender Oil
- 1 tsp — Glycerin
- 3 tbsp — Aloe Vera Gel

Gently combine all ingredients until well blended.

Pour into your favorite dispenser container – pumps work well with this mixture.

Apply whenever a gently hand wash is needed without water.

Moisture Infusing Waterless Hand Wash
Antibacterial/Moisturizing

This is a great waterless wash I like to carry in my purse. The recipe provides a mild anti-bacterial effect while providing moisture throughout the day. I use this not only when I need to clean my hands but whenever I want a light moisture benefit on the road.

- ¼ tsp   Borax Powder

- 4 tbsp   Rosewater

- 2 tbsp   Glycerin

- ¼ cup   Aloe Vera Gel

Heat rosewater and glycerin in a microwave safe dish for 45 seconds

Dissolve borax mixture into heated liquid. Stir gently to prevent foaming.

Slowly pour mixture into aloe base and stir until all ingredients are well blended.

Pour into your favorite applicator container – this mixture also pumps well.

Moisturizing Antibacterial Liquid Soap

We keep this soap on the kitchen sink year round since it is a light cleanser that combines a mild anti-bacterial effect with a very gentle cleansing.

- ➤ ½ cup   Castile Soap

- ➤ 1/8 cup   Honey

- ➤ 1 tbsp   Fresh Lemon Juice

- ➤ 3 drops   Tincture of Benzoin

Mix all ingredients until well blended.

Pour into your favorite applicator bottle.

This is a soap mixture so always rinse hands thoroughly when done washing.

Castile soap can be made at home following the basic recipe in the soap making section.

Foaming Anti-bacterial Scrub

When I have been working around the house or garden and my hands are especially dirty a foaming wash makes me feel cleaner. This combines a gently cleansing agent with anti-bacterial benefits in a great foamy wash.

- ➤ 3 tbsp   Coconut Oil

- ➤ 1 tsp   Grapefruit Juice

- ➤ 1 tsp   Honey

- ➤ 3 tbsp   Witch Hazel

- ➤ ¼ tsp   Tincture of Benzoin

- ➤ 1 crushed   Vitamin C Tablet

Dissolve the Vitamin C powder in the witch hazel mixture.

Blend remaining ingredients.

Stir gently until well blended.

Mixture will foam if stirred too vigorously.

Pour into your favorite applicator container and use as a soap as desired.

Softening Anti bacterial Lotion

At times my hands become very dried and unattractive from the too frequent washings so I try to use an anti-bacterial lotion in place of a wash as often as possible. This is a great lotion I keep in both the kitchen and bath to rub into my hands.

- ➢ 1/8 cup   Cocoa Butter (tub form)

- ➢ 4 tbsp   Lemon Juice

- ➢ 2 tbsp   Zinc Oxide

- ➢ 3 tbsp   Lecithin

Blend all ingredients and store tightly sealed container.

Apply to hands and other body parts as desired.

This will form a thicker protective coating on the hands while delivering a mild antibacterial benefit and softening the skin.

Deodorant

All deodorants share two common goals. To help you control perspiration and to aid you in feeling fresh and clean. Perspiration itself is odorless, but when the bacteria on the surface of your skin react with perspiration the two components create body odor. We are all familiar with body odor and it is not a pleasant smell. This is the reason anti-perspirant products are a staple in each of our medicine cabinets.

There are two main types of products that aid you in the prevention of body odor, Antiperspirants and Deodorants.

➤ An antiperspirant contains astringent products. An astringent reduces the size of the pores of your body and helps to limit the amount of perspiration that your body produces.

➤ Deodorants contain antibacterial agents that kill the bacteria on the surface of your skin while adding a pleasing scent.

Some people prefer to use an antiperspirant alone. This helps to limit the odor causing bacteria while allowing the body to produce perspiration naturally. Antiperspirant actually tightens the body's pores and limits the amount of perspiration released.

A deodorant kills odor causing bacteria on the surface of the skin. A deodorant does not interfere with the body's natural perspiration processes.

Other people use a combination product that limits the perspiration produced, kills the odor causing bacteria, and provides a fresh scent. These combination products are popular in the marketplace today and provide the benefits and protections of both core ingredients.

When choosing the type of products you wish to create and use you will want to understand the basic biological facts behind perspiration.

Perspiration helps the body regulate its temperature. It also serves to release excess salts and toxic substances from the body. Fresh perspiration is odorless. The bacterium on the skin surface reacts with the perspiration to cause body odor. Therefore, for some people, simply limiting the amount of bacteria on the skin surface may provide enough protection while others may need to limit the amount of perspiration the body produces.

Each person's body chemistry is slightly different and different recipes and ingredients will work better for one person then another. You should experiment with a variety of recipes and ingredients to determine which products will work best for you.

You will also need to decide how you prefer to apply your product. People with sensitive skin may prefer cream style products while others may prefer stick style or even spray style products. Each of these recipes can be modified to obtain the preferred method of application that suits you the best.

We have included some basic recipes to get you started. You will want to review the ingredients listing very carefully to determine which other natural anti-bacterial products might work best for you and which might not work for you and your family.

Cream Deodorant

This is an excellent cream deodorant. This form of deodorant works well for people with sensitive skin as it is not as harsh or as drying as the spray forms. I like to use this deodorant in the winter months when my skin is already somewhat dry. The use of the cocoa butter provides a moisturizing, protective coating that aids in conditioning and protecting the sensitive skin areas.

- ¼ c   Cocoa Butter

- 1 tbsp.   Cornstarch Powder

- 2 tsp.   Baking Soda

- 1 tsp.   Liquid Chlorophyll

- ¼ tsp.   incture of Benzoin

- ¼ tsp.   Stearic acid

- *Fragrance, Color, Emulsifier & Thickener as desired*

Place all ingredients in a plastic or wooden mixing bowl.

Stir well using a plastic utensil (not metal).

Spoon cream mixture into your favorite clean container and seal tightly.

Apply using a cotton ball or clean cloth.

Alum Powder may be added for antiperspirant qualities. Be sure to use only USP Grade for Cosmetic use Alum Powder.

This recipe will have a lovely green color but if you desire a specific color or fragrance you may add your favorite food coloring or essential oils to the recipe to obtain a customized appearance.

All Over Deodorant Powder

This is an excellent odor reducing powder that is an effective moisture absorber for any area of the body. I make a few jars of this powder with different scents for use on different areas of my body.

- ½ cup   Cornstarch Powder

- 2 tbsp.   Baking Soda

- 1 tsp.   Liquid Chlorophyll

- *Fragrance, Color, Emulsifier & Thickener as desired*

Place all ingredients in a jar and shake until chlorophyll is evenly dispersed.

A jar with shaker slots on the top works best.

Simply wipe or shake on area desired for a smooth, fresh feeling.

The finished powder will have a pretty green color but if you desire a specific color or fragrance you may add your favorite food coloring or essential oils to the recipe to obtain a customized appearance.

Witch Hazel Spray

This is an excellent deodorant spray that will leave you feeling invigorated and refreshed. It works especially well for sensitive skin or irritated areas. I often use this spray after shaving because it has a soothing effect on the shaved areas. The witch hazel provides a refreshing, soothing action while the honey provides an anti-bacterial, protective coating. Alum powder is a natural astringent making this product an excellent combination product. Be sure to use only USP Grade for Cosmetic use Alum Powder.

> ➢ 1 cup   Water

> ➢ ¼ cup   Witch Hazel

> ➢ 2 tsp.   Alum Powder

> ➢ 1 tsp.   Honey

> ➢   *Fragrance, Color, Emulsifier & Thickener as desired*

You may add your favorite color or essential oils to the mixture to give the deodorant a customized scent that suits your daily care ritual.

Combine all ingredients in a clean plastic spray container (do not use metal) and shake well to mix.

You may want to shake this before each application to ensure proper mixing.

Spray on desired area daily for a clean fresh feeling.

Makes approximately 1 ¼ cup spray

Lemon Spray

This recipe is an effective anti-perspirant and deodorant spray that works well in the warmer months. The addition of lemon and honey provide extra anti-bacterial properties while the lemon gives a refreshing scent suitable for either men or women.

- ➢ 1 cup Water
- ➢ 1 ½ tsp.   Alum Powder
- ➢ ¼ cup   Vodka
- ➢ 2 tbsp.   Lemon Juice
- ➢ 1 tbsp. Baking Soda
- ➢ 1 tsp.   Honey
- ➢   *Fragrance, Color, Emulsifier & Thickener as desired*

This may be sticky when you first make it. The stickiness will abate as the product ages. I like to set it aside for about a week before use but you can use it right away if you wish.

Dissolve alum powder and baking soda in water in a plastic or ceramic container (do not use metal).

Be sure to use only USP Grade for Cosmetic use Alum Powder.

Add the remaining ingredients and stir or shake to mix well.

Pour into a spray bottle and apply daily.

This mixture will have a lovely pale gold color and the light scent of lemons, but if you desire a specific color or fragrance you may add your favorite food coloring or essential oils to the recipe to obtain a customized appearance.

Makes approximately 1 ½ cups spray.

Baking Soda Sensitive Skin Deodorant

This is an effective deodorant for people with sensitive skin. The baking soda and cornstarch provide soothing odor absorbing components while the beeswax provides anti-bacterial skin protection. The addition of alum powder makes this a natural antiperspirant.

- ¼ cup   Grated Beeswax
- 2 tbsp.   Petroleum Jelly

Heat beeswax and jelly approximately 45 seconds in microwave safe dish until beeswax is a golden liquid color. Allow to cool slightly.

- 3 tbsp.   Cornstarch Powder
- 2 tbsp.   Baking Soda
- 2 tbsp.   Alum Powder

Gently stir the dry ingredients with a plastic spoon being sure all ingredients are well blended.

Be sure to use only USP Grade for Cosmetic use Alum Powder.

Pour the mixture into a greased plastic or ceramic dish and allow to harden.

Cut the mixture into cakes and apply.

You may add your favorite sent or essential oils to the mixture to give the deodorant a customized scent that suits your daily care ritual.

Basic Anti-Perspirant Spray

This is an excellent spray which will act as an anti-perspirant only. This is an especially popular spray for men.

- ➤ 1 ½ tsp.   Alum Powder

- ➤ ¼ c   Witch Hazel

- ➤ ½ cup   Water

Be sure to use only USP Grade for Cosmetic use Alum Powder.

If you desire a specific color or fragrance you may add your favorite food coloring or essential oils to the recipe to obtain a customized appearance.

Combine all ingredients in a plastic spray container and shake well to mix.

Spray on desired area daily for a clean fresh feeling.

You may want to shake this mixture before each application to ensure the ingredients are well mixed.

Makes approximately 3/4 cup spray

Citrus Anti-perspirant/Deodorant Spray

This recipe is an effective anti-perspirant and deodorant spray that works well in the warmer months. The lemon provides a fresh citrus and combined with the baking soda provides extra odor absorption protection. The alum powder acts as a natural anti-perspirant. This spray is effective for men or woman and can be customized by adding a favorite scent.

- ➤ 1 cup   Water

- ➤ 1 ½ tsp.   Alum Powder

- ➤ ¼ cup   Vodka

- ➤ 2 tbsp.   Lemon Juice

- ➤ 1 tbsp.   Baking Soda

Dissolve alum powder and baking soda in water.

Use only plastic or ceramic bowls and utensils.

Use only USP Grade for Cosmetic use Alum Powder.

Add the remaining ingredients and shake to mix well.

This mixture will have a very pale yellow color and the light scent of lemon, but if you desire a specific color or fragrance you may add your favorite food coloring or essential oils to the recipe to obtain a customized appearance.

Pour into a spray bottle and apply daily.

You may want to shake this mixture before each application to ensure all ingredients are well mixed.

Make approximately 1 ½ cups spray.

Heat Wave Spray

I love this mixture during the hottest times of the year. I also spritz this combination on my face, neck, and arms during the warmer months for a quick refresher throughout the day.

> 2 tsp   Glycerin

> ¼ cup   Witch Hazel

> ¼ tsp   Liquid Chlorophyll

> 1 tsp   Alum Powder

> 2 tsp   Pineapple Juice

Mix all ingredients in a plastic or ceramic container (do not use metal).

Use only USP Grade for Cosmetic use Alum Powder.

This mixture will be a light green color and have a sweet fragrance but if you desire a specific color or fragrance you may add your favorite food coloring or essential oils to the recipe to obtain a customized appearance.

Allow mixture to sit in a cool location for 10-12 days to ensure all ingredients activate properly and to minimize some of the sticky sensation that can be present immediately after mixing.

This mixture works best if you store in the refrigerator.

To apply spray on desired area or apply with a cotton ball or clean cloth

Appendix A
Ingredient List

All natural make up and personal care products have become 'the thing' for many people. Whether from a desire to reduce chemical usage, reduce expenses, address specific issues better than the mass market products or just live a more natural life, more and more people I speak with are making their own cleaners, make-up and beauty products.

My family has used 'natural' products for years. My mother and grandmother both had skin and allergy issues and passed many home cleaning, personal care, and other product ideas down to my daughter and I. My daughter was born with the same sensitive skin and had the added issue of being a chemical reactive asthmatic.

I have posted many video and recipe instructions for the products that we use and enjoy the most. However, there are many reasons that people want to make their own natural products and your needs may not be the same as ours. There are also many combinations of product components that we have not yet tried. The following pages list some of the most commonly used elements and their supposed properties and effects.

Before you begin using the included ingredient lists, please remember that the properties and effects shown for each ingredient has not been fully proven and in many cases endorsed by the FDA or AMA. Whenever I am aware of a particular approval or endorsement, have included the information. All of this information has been gathered over years of use, chats with other people, and trial and error research. Please use your care and your own common sense when trying any of the included ingredients.

Enjoy!

Acacia	Powdered Acacia is used as a binding agent for lotions, ointments, and other liquids to semi-solids Soluble in cold water Improves texture of semi-solid preparations
Acetamide MEA	Used as a stabilizer
AHA	Alpha Hydroxyl Acids are acids extracted from fruit, sugar and vegan lactic acid Will dissolve dead cells Mild peeling and moisturizing Use 1 – 5% in creams and gels DO NOT use around eyes or on sensitive skin
Almond Oil	Easily absorbed Natural astringent and emollient characteristics Softens and conditions the skin and hair Used in lotions, treatments, and ointments For all skin types Alleviate itchy skin conditions
Alkanet Root	Red root that comes from a tree Aids in the dying of products
Allantoin Powder	Protects against harsher components of recipes Helps stimulate growth of tissues Use .5 to 2% in creams Inhibits allergic responses Dissolve in a little cold water and then add while product is less than 40 degrees Classified by the Food and Drug Administration (FDA) Over-The-Counter (OTC) Topical Analgesic review Panel as a Category I (safe and effective) active

ingredient skin protect, at use-levels of 0.5 - 2.0%. FDA approved applications include minor cuts, scrapes, burns, sunburn, fever blisters, diaper rash and chaffed, chapped, cracked or wind burned skin and lips. It is a skin protect for use in creams, lotions, lip products, shaving creams, suntan products, scalp healing products, and baby products Reference FDA Release

Almond Butter

Excellent spreadability
Adds moisturizing attributes to creams, lotions, bar soaps, hair care, sun care, balms and oils

Almond Oil

Contains Oleic Acid, fatty acids, sterolins and Vitamin E
Nearly odorless
Skin nutrition
Similar to skins natural oil
Natural emollient
Tames fly away
For all skin & hair types

Aloe, Aloe Vera

Soothing
Anti-inflammatory
Antibacterial
Treatment of acne
Highly emollient
Believed to stimulate collagen synthesis and skin regeneration
Leaf is rubbed on dry hair tame fly away ends
Oil promotes healing and replaces lost moisture
Improves hydration
Cuticle – heals, smoothes, softens

Aloe Butter

Extract of aloe in a coconut base
Solid at room temp but melts on the skin
Lotions & creams 3-5%, Balms 5-100%,
Conditioners 2-5%

Aloe Oil

Add healing properties to recipes without
bacterial or mold growth (5-10%)

Aloe Wood

Used in skin tonic mixtures
May have pigment restoration qualities

Alpha Hydroxyl Acids(AHA)

Mild acids that remove the outer layer of
dull skin
Creates a rejuvenated appearance
Contains glycolic, lactic, malic, citric and
tartaric acids that are mild acids used to
remove the outer layer of dull skin
From citrus fruits, apples and grapes
Glycolic acid is found in sugar cane
Lactic acid is found in milk
The FDA now requires that any product
containing AHA's have the following
warning statement: This product contains
an alpha hydroxyl acid (AHA) that may
increase your skin's sensitivity to the sun
and particularly the possibility of sunburn.
Use a sunscreen and limit sun exposure
while using this product and for a week
afterwards
Reference: FDA Release

Aluminum Sulfate

Acts as an antiseptic
Aids in stopping bleeding
Aids in tightening skin
Tightening agent for year rounds use in
aging products
*** Purchase ONLY cosmetic grade

Amino Acids - Oat

Oat Amino Acids penetrate easily
Humectants, soothing, itch reliever,
moisturizer
Deposit protective film on hair –
smoothing and moisturizing

Amino Acids - Silk

Body uses as a building block
Penetrates well

Ammonium Lauryl
Sulphate

Shampoo base derived from coconuts
Creates lather
Cleanses hair while separating strands to
give volume
Promotes spreading of product

Andiroba Oil

The oil contains myristic acid
Help minimize the growth of the pigment
producing cells that cause age spots

Apache Plume

Root and bark are boiled as with tea
Used as a hair tonic to promote growth

Apple Juice

From the apple
Rich in pectin

Apricot Kernel Oil

From apricot pits
Similar to natural oils
Moisture without oily film
Rich in Vitamin A
Extremely nourishing
Emollient
Softer and smoother feel
Easily absorbed by the hair and skin
Infuses moisture into the hair and skin

Argan Oil

Helps increase squalene
Rich in Vitamin E and Fatty Acids
Absorbs Quickly
Strengthens Brittle Hair & Nails

	Believed to replace lost moisture Anti-aging effect when massaged into the skin
Arrowroot	Minor anesthetic qualities Excellent balm for irritated scalp Thickening and stabilizing agent
Ascorbyl Palmitate	Palmitic acid ester - Vitamin C Ester Salt of ascorbic acid Used as a preservative and antioxidant Believed to remove the free radicals that cells produce
Asphodelus	Used as part of a topical ointment or cream to fade freckles, age spots, scar tissue, and excess skin pigmentation
Avocado	From the fruit of avocados Used often as a moisturizer Protects hair and skin in hot, dry climates Rich in oils Sunscreen properties NOT for oily skin Year round uses especially in summer Nail – Cuticle care Rich in Vitamins B, E, and K Deep moisture treatments
Avocado Butter	Soft greenish butter Mild odor but excellent melting properties Softens and moisturizes
Avocado Oil	Rich, heavy, penetrating oil Vitamin A, C, D, E NOT for oily skin May repel UV rays DILUTE with other oils to minimize thickness
Baking Soda	Clarifying agent

	Softens water to enable cleaning agents to work better
Bananas	Mashed fruit of the banana Rich in oils Non-irritating Excellent for all hair types High potassium content makes it difficult for bacteria to survive Rich in Vitamin A
Bay Rum	Stimulates scalp to encourage hair growth
Bearsfoot Root/ Yellow Leaf Cup root	Used as an ointment Shampoo component to treat scalp conditions such as dandruff
Beer	Beer is an excellent product base for hair rinse or finishing products The sugar base and protein components of the beer act as a thickening agent and can be used as a hair rinse or combed through hair before styling to provide a fuller, lustrous look to the hair Aroma fades as beer dries Hair – especially for thinning or fine hair Thickens, adds shine, and adds bounce Rinse or styling agent Year round use
Beet-root Powder Beet Juice	Purple red color Tastes sweet
Benzoin	Use benzoin resin in external skin applications heal cuts, sooth inflammation of rough cracked skin Used as a preservative in cosmetics and a fixative for perfume

Beta carotene	Vitamin A Found in plants and many animal tissues Has an orange pigment and is used as a coloring agent in several cosmetics Excessive beta carotene in the blood can lead to a yellow-red pigmentation of the skin
Birch bark	Helps halt hair loss
Black Seed Oil	Nutrating oil Contains fatty oils, vitamins & minerals May aid in preventing hair loss Contains amino acids that help to strengthen and nourish the hair May combat alopecia when included in a topical scalp treatment
Borage	High gamma linolenic acid GLA – Vitamin for skin Humectants Skin disorders like psoriasis and eczema, and sun damaged or aged skin Regenerating and stimulating for all skin types
Borax	Used as a preservative and texturizer Excellent cleanser that is mild and allows the creation of cleansing products without drying the skin and hair Adds foaming effect to soaps ** Borax Powder (Sodium Borate – natural source of cosmetic grade borax that does not contain surfactants and detergents. Acts as an emulsifier
Burdock Root Oil	Also known as Bur Oil Improves hair strength, shine & body

May help prevent hair loss
Soothing – eases dandruff & scalp itching
Promotes hair strength, shine, and body
Boil ½ tsp of root in 1 cup of water and allow to steep for 30 minutes. Up to 3 x's daily.
Burdock root tea can be used alone or as a part of a skin wash to help combat acne

Cajeput	Astringent oil Good for oily skin Helps clear eczema
Calendula Oil	Targets oil or Marigold Oil Antiseptic, antifungal, anti-inflammatory Healing, soothing – all skin types Can relieve acne
Camphor	Antibacterial, astringent Combat oily skin and acne
Cantaloupe	Light hair conditioner for oily hair
Carmine	Red pigment derived from dried cochineal Excellent dye for lipsticks
Carrot Oil	Rich in beta carotene, Vitamin A & E Balance moisture in skin and conditions hair Revitalizes and tones and nourishes skin Easily absorbed Helps balance both oily and dry complexions Heals damaged skin Helps aged skin
Castile Soap	Made from olive oil

Extremely mild, liquid with water-like
consistency
Can be used on both hair and skin
Provides gentle cleansing without drying
Leaves a soft, moist feel when rinsed

Castor Oil   Hard shiny oil that acts as a barrier agent
                      and protector
                      Found in many cosmetics

Cedar wood   Sedative, astringent, antiseptic
                      Used to treat oily skin and scalp
                      Relieve itching, psoriasis, eczema,
                      High concentrations will irritate the skin
                      Good insect repellent - mosquitoes,
                      moths, woodworms, leeches and rats

Centaury   Helps clear blemishes
                      Softens the skin
                      Said to remove freckles, age, & hyper-
                      pigmentation

Cetearyl Alcohol   Emulsifying wax produced from mixture of
                      fatty alcohols
                      Forms a barrier film to keep moisture from
                      evaporating
                      Give hair and skin a velvety feeling
                      Used to add body and compatibility to
                      hair

Cetearyl Glycoside   Made of glucose and cetearyl alcohol
                      Helps hair retain moisture
                      Creates velvety feeling

Champagne   Can also use sparkling wine
                      Rich in sugars and proteins
                      Acts much like beer and thickens hair
                      while providing body and bounce.
                      Hair – Styling lotion, thickening rinse,

wet/dry gel
Promotes tissue regeneration
Used to treat dermatitis, minor skin
irritation and inflammation
Bleaches fine, light hair

Clary Sage

Treatment for oily hair and skin
Dandruff control treatment
Treats wrinkles

Chlorophyll

Derived from the leaves of green plant
Promotes healing
Excellent deodorizer

Cinnamon

Darkens hair

Citric Acid

Preservative
Extends products shelf life
Helps products retain texture and guards
against appearance loss
Blends easily
Contains Alpha Hydroxyl

Cleavers

Used as a skin wash
Improve complexion
Treats skin disorders
Used as a dandruff relief hair rinse

Cocomphcaroxy-
glycinate

From coconuts
Works with sodium lauryl sulphate
Makes shampoo milder on skin and hair

Cocomide DEA

From coconuts
Makes bubbles smaller so that foam is
thicker and richer
Fatty acid from coconut oil and glycerin
Used in shampoos, conditioners and
shower gels as a thickener and foamier

Cocoamidopropyl Betaine	A coconut oil compound Used as an emulsifier, thickener, foam booster, and conditioner
Cocoa Butter	Soften and lubricate Cuticles – soften/protects Hair – styling tames hair on ends – similar to wax works Prevents drying and chapping 100% COCOA BUTTER ONLY
Coconut Oil	From coconuts Provides exceptional protective layer to hair, skin, lips, and cuticles Locks in moisture Straighten hair while locking in moisture Emollient Treats dry, damaged hair Suitable for all skin and hair Penetrates into the deeper layers of the skin to helping to keep connective tissues strong and supple Easily absorbed Helps to reduce the appearance of fine lines and wrinkles Aid in exfoliating the outer layer of dead skin cells
Cod Liver Oil	Source of EPA and DHA and Vitamin A&D
Collagen	Pseudo Collagen Derived from yeast Mimics the action of collagen and confers moisture Binding Adds body and shine to hair Pour. 5 to 10% into product while under 40 degrees

Copaiba	Effective in fighting dandruff Relieve inflammation Help heal athlete's foot, eczema and psoriasis, Heals damaged skin with minimal scarring
Cornflower	Astringent Added to shampoo to treat eczema of the scalp
Cornstarch	From corn ground fine – white powder Replaces many powder ingredients Excellent thickening agent Absorbs Moisture & Oils Leaves hair extra shiny
Cottonseed Oil	Rich in Vitamin E
Cranberry Seed Oil	Skin, hair, lips and baby care Contributes to lipid barrier protection Assists in moisture retention
Cypress	Reduces excess oils in skin and hair care products Tightens skin Refine the appearance of pores Reduces excess sweating in overly oily hair
Diazolidinyl Urea	Preservative
Distilled Water	Water with all minerals, bacteria and other substances removed
Egg Yolks	Contains lecithin - a natural emulsifier and preservative Rick in protein Aids in creating shiny, thicker hair Hair – deep conditioner, hair thickening

agent
NOT moisturizing
Excellent for oily hair

Elderberry	Darkens gray hair
Emulsifier	Used to create bond between water and oil Critical in lotions and creams Makes a fluid cream and lotion without separation Nice end texture Mixes two opposing liquids making it an excellent additive for many products
Evening Primrose Oil	Nutrating oil Contains fatty oils, vitamins & minerals May aid in preventing hair loss AMA says makes skin softer, smoother, reduces roughness, cracking and irritation Reference AMA Release
Flax Oil	Richest source of alpha linolenic acid Reduces trans epidermal water loss from skin
Fumitory	Treatment for eczema and other eruptions of the skin Helps removing freckles
Gelatin	Derived from animal collagen Beneficial to hair and nails Contains high levels of sugar and protein Help repair damaged hair and promote body Setting agent or deep conditioner for hair Can be used as a rub for nails
Germall Plus	Preservative

Liquid / water soluble
Highly effective

Geranium	Mature and troubled skin care Creates a radiant glow
Ginkgo	Improves circulation aiding in combating hair loss
Glycerin	Natural humectants (attracts and holds moisture) Pulls oxygen from air and brings it to hair Very gentle even for sensitive skin Year round use for hair Perfect for all weather Vegetable glycerin – natural emollient Hypoallergenic
Gotu kola	Contains asiaticoside Works to stimulate skin repair Strengthens skin, hair, nails, and connective tissue
Grapefruit Juice	High in citric acid Contains natural sugars, which help thicken and hold hair in place OILY hair only Hair – Oily hair styling agent, Hair Spray
Grapefruit Oil	Hair growth Antiseptic, Astringent Oily hair only
Grapefruit Seed Oil	Made from dried ground seeds and pulp of grapefruit Natural preservative Antiseptic, anti bacterial Stabilizing for most products Combined with glycerin in many items

Pippen

Grapeseed Oil
Odorless oil
Base for many creams, lotions and as a carrier oil
Does not leave greasy feeling
Non-allergenic
Oleic, linolec, palmitric and stearic acids
Emollient and toning to all skin types

Green Tea Extract
From the leaves of the plan dried, cured, extracted into ethyl alcohol
Astringent
Mixes well with both oil and water based products

Guar Gum
Made from the ground seed tissue of plants
Used as a thickener
Has 5 to 8 times the thickening properties of starch

Hazelnut Oil
High in Vitamin E
Easily absorbed into hair

Hempseed Oil
Highly absorbent, soothing
Especially rich oil
Said to stimulate cell growth
High in linolenic acid
Emollient
AMA – skin feel softer, smoother, reduce roughness, cracking and irritation
May retard fine wrinkles of aging
hair care products, hemp seed oil increases elasticity, manageability, and shine
Reference AMA

Henna Leaves
From henna plants these leaves are resinous

171

Provides a protective coating for hair, lips, nails and skin
Can be used colored in tanning products and hair dyes
Locks in moisture
Protects from elements
*** Henna is a dye – colorless leaves are available.
Purchase only 100% henna at most drugstores and pharmacies
Nails – strengthening agent
Locks in moisture
Excellent for dry, damaged, weak nails
Hair – provides a thicker, lustrous appearance for hair
Locks in moisture, protects and strengths

Hibiscus Flowers   Provides red highlights to light or dark hair

Honey   Derived from the nectar of flowers and plants and created by bees as a by-product of honeycomb creation
98% sugar and 2% enzymes
Full of Vitamins and minerals
Has a stimulating and toning effect
Natural humectants
High potassium content inhibits bacteria growth
Excellent component for moisturizing formulations
The DARKER the honey the better the effect care because the dark honey contains more minerals.
Attracts moisture and helps lock it in place
Hydrates
*** Do not use honey in child care products or those who commonly come into contact with children as honey can

be harmful to the very young
*** Natural preservative
Lips/nails – harsh climatic conditions –
attracts and holds moisture
Hair – humectants which attracts and
holds moisture. Assist in curly hair curl hold
Hair – lightens slightly – use molasses for
darker hair care products

Honey Powder

Full of Vitamins and minerals
Natural humectants
High potassium content inhibits bacteria
growth
Excellent component for moisturizing
formulations
*** Do not use honey in child care
products or those who commonly come
into contact with children as honey can
be harmful to the very young
*** Natural preservative

Imidazolidinyl Urea

Preservative

Immortelle

Stimulate the production of new skin cells
Mature skin products

Jasmine

Used in ointments for dry sensitive skin

Jojoba Oil

Actually a liquid wax
Very similar to body's natural oil making it
easily absorbed
Perfect for any moisturizing agent
Will solidify if kept cold
Mimics collagen
Year round use for hair, nails, skin and lips
Moisture – hair and skin easily absorbed
Natural preservative
Carrier oil
Scalp cleanser for hair

(application) 11%
Hypoallergenic and pure

Kokum Butter

Naturally white and very smooth
Emollient properties
Hard / solid – melts on contact
Lotions and creams 1-3%, balms 5-100%,
conditioners 1-3%

Kukui Nut Oil

Expressed from the nuts, and is light yellow
with an amber tint
Aids in softening and restructuring
Easily absorbed
Highly penetrating
Hydrate and soften

Lanolin Oil

From glands of sheep
Waxy feel substance
Acts as moisturizing agent for skin, lips,
nails
Setting lotion for hair
Helps absorb and retain moisture
May penetrate the skin and hair follicles
Deep treatment base
Deep conditioning
Emollient – soothing and softening

Lavender Oil

From lavender flowers
Antiseptic – germ killing properties
Enhances highlights in dark hair and
darkens lighter hair
Astringent - ideal for oily and combination
skin

Lauramide DEA

From coconut and palm kernel oils
Prevents harsh stripping action of
shampoo by coating hair and giving
bounce

Lauryl Betaine	From coconut and palm kernel oils Boost foam in shampoo
Lecithin	Derived from egg yolks , soybeans, and corn A natural emollient Allow special proteins to penetrate better Attracts water from the air and holds hydration in place – skin and hair. Can get in powder form Emulsifier and thickening agent
Lemon Balm	Baldness Prevention
Lemon / Citrus	Derived from the juice of citrus fruits Anti-bacterial Creates highlights in light hair when used in small quantity in a hair rinse Hair – year round use as a clarifying agent to reduce the build up of gels and oils *** Remember lightening effect – dark hair use Baking Soda
Lemongrass	Astringent, anti-septic, anti-infectious, antifungal Good for oily hair Reduces excessive sweating and enlarged pores Great for oily skin and hair
Lemon Oil	Balances sebum (skin oil) Increases shine and growth of hair and nails Astringent Lightens hair Brighten dull complexions Gentle cleanser for oily skin and hair Acne treatments Add after any steps that require heat

Do not expose to high temperatures

Macadamia Nut Oil	Similar to sebum (natural oil) Absorbs well Emollient and soother
Magnesium Sulfate	Water softener
Magnesium Stearate	From ester of magnesium and stearic acid Odorless fine white powder Soluble in warm alcohol Insoluble but dispersible in water and oils Provides opacity, texture & consistency
Mayonnaise	Created from eggs, oil and vinegar Moisturizing agent for hair Oil and eggs provide nourishment for hair and skin The vinegar provides a clarifying effect to hair and skin Can be used as a deep moisturizing agent
Meadow foam Seed	Adds shine and moisture to hair and scalp Helps dry and brittle hair Cuticle repair, body oils, shaving creams
Menthol Paraben	Non-toxic, nonirritating Preservative Stable in most ingredients – water soluble
Milk, Goat	Lactose leaves the hair and skin feeling silky smooth Softening cleanser Hydrates Alpha hydroxyl treatments = lactic acid (milk) + citric acid, glycolic, malic and tartaric acids

Milk, Powdered	Lactose leaves the hair and skin feeling silky smooth Excellent softening cleanser Hydrates Alpha hydroxyl treatments = lactic acid (milk) + citric acid, glycolic, malic and tartaric acids.
Mint Leaves	Rich in iron Natural energizer Kills bacteria
Nettle Leaves / Root	Stimulates hair growth Improve condition of scalp Contains chlorophyll and silicone - silicone assists in hair and nail strength
Oats	Oatmeal Soothing skin treatment - dry skin, sunburns, eczema, psoriasis
Olive Leaf	Relieve itchy scalp
Olive Oil	Nutritive and stable Superior penetrating power Acidic and antioxidant Cleaning agent shampoo/conditioner
Optiphen	Liquid preservative Add at anytime during creation
Orange Flower Water	Derived from orange blossoms Astringent and cleanser Hair – remove gel and build-up
Orange Peel	Use the entire orange peel (white and orange)

	Mild abrasive combined with the natural solvent of orange oils Vitamin rich
Orrisroot	Derived from root of white iris Used as fixative for perfumes and powders Retains aromas
Palm Kernel Oil	Similar to coconut oil Lathers well
Papaya Paw Paw	Natural softener for hair and skin Creates a velvety feel
Patchouli	Heals dry and itching skin
Pear Juice	Good source of sorbitol – humectants Attracts moisture Provides a smooth texture Assists in curl creation Apples, cherries, plums and berries have the same effect
Pineapple Juice	Contains bromalain, a protein digesting enzyme Removes dead cells, surface dirt, and oils Hair – clarifying treatment for oily hair
Polysorbate 20	Vicious oily liquid from lauric acid Emulsifier Common component of coconut oil Allows water to penetrate more easily
Pomegranate	Use only the seeds, not the whole fruit Deep penetrating oil High in flavinoids Good for dry, devitalized skin Aids in moisturizing skin, preventing and

reducing the appearance of wrinkles
Used to treat dry skin, eczema, psoriasis

Proteins

Add gloss, body and luster to hair
Plant proteins have excellent skin
compatibility

Propyl Glycol

From lactic acid, glucose or seaweed
Most common moisture carrying agent in
cosmetics
Moisturizes better than glycerin
Gives product better absorption and
spreadability
AMA says – safe in cosmetics

Propyl Paraben

Widely used in cosmetics
Preservative against bacteria and fungus
Paraben is neutral – non irritating, non-
sensitizing

Psyllium Seeds

From plants
These create a very thick gel
Surrounds hair and helps hold a set
Tames fly away hair and for structured
styles

Pygeum

Used with Saw Palmetto & Stinging Nettle
Root for hair loss treatments

Red Raspberry Oil

UV absorptive properties – all three levels

Rhubarb

Lightens hair
Mix w/ shampoo for color treatment

Rose / Rose Water

Astringent skin care wash
Speeds healing

Rosehip Seed Oil

Derived from the ripened fruit of a hybrid
rosebush

Strengthens hair shaft
AMA says it makes skin feel softer and
smoother, reduce roughness, cracking
and irritation. Possibly retard the fine
wrinkles of aging
Reference AMA Release

Rosemary Oil

Antioxidant
More stable than Vitamin E for products
and creams
Helps stop products from going rancid
Preservative
Tames fly away hair
Brings out warmth in darker hair
Stimulates the scalp
Slows hair loss
Speeds hair growth
Astringent
Anti-bacterial

Safflower Oil

Highest Linoleic Acid
Moisturizing
Treats dry and damaged skin
Soothing to skin
Contains two colorants – yellow & red
Used for dyeing silk
Mixed with finely-powdered was used to
create rouge.'
Pale yellow oils contain proteins, minerals,
vitamins
Good for all skin types

Sage

Darkening Hair Dye - Especially for gray
hair
Stimulating to the scalp
Softens & shines hair
Invigorates scalp
Dries perspiration – lessens body odor
Oils are antiseptic and antibiotic

Sal Butter	Stable Extremely emollient Prevents drying Directly applied in solid state or mixed
Sandalwood	Relieves inflammation and itching Helps dry and dehydrated skin Mild astringent Helps with acne and other inflammatory skin conditions Good for oily skin
Saw Palmetto	Saw palmetto inhibits dihydotestosterone (DHT), - enzyme that is associated with male pattern baldness May halt hair loss Stimulates healthy hair growth
Sea Buckthorn	Combat wrinkles Good for severe dryness Used as part of treatment for premature aging Repairs, conditions, and heals damaged skin Acne treatment Will stain skin, surfaces and clothing. Apply evenly to skin surfaces Dilute prior to use Use at room temperature
Sea Silk	Marine vegetable Provides protein enrichment Creates silky feeling Protective, moisturizing film Soothes the scalp 2-3% into product while under 40 degrees
Seaweed	Contains carregenall which is an

emulsifier

Sesame Oil	From sesame seeds Sunscreen One of the deepest natural oils
Shea butter	Rich is vitamins A, E, and F Protects the skin from free radicals Helps prevent lines and wrinkles Moisturizes dry, heat-damaged, over processed hair. Hydrates hair Humectants - draws moisture into the hair Coats the shaft to make hair soft Forms breathable, water resistant film Compatible with all hair types Solid Melts at skin temp Use as little heat as possible to reduce granules 3-5% lotions and creams, 5-100% balms, 3-6% bar soaps, 2-5% conditioners
Slippery Elm	Emollient Slightly astringent
Soapwort	Base ingredient in liquid soap, shampoo, & conditioner Not lathering Gives hair & skin a slippery feel
Sodium Hydroxymethylglycinate	Antimicrobial Used in VERY low concentrations Preservative for products – can be used in place of TEA Active regardless of the other ingredients used in the recipe Amino acid – helps penetration

Sodium Lauryl Sulfoacetate	Free flowing white powder Use in cream and paste shampoos, cleansing creams, and bars Provides foaming and viscosity Milder to the skin than ethoxylated alcohol sulfates such as Sodium Lauryl Sulfate Hard water stable Used to replace soap 3% concentration
Sodium Laureth	Shampoo base from palm and coconut oils Foams and cleanses
Sorbitol	Humectants Gives smooth feel to hair Used instead of glycerin in many recipes Occurs in ripe berries, cherries, plums, pears, apples, seaweed, and algae Humectrant and a binder Gives hair and skin a velvety feel
Soyamidopropl Betaine	Compound from soybean oil & alcohol Used as an emulsifier, thickener, foam booster and conditioner
Spearmint	May help to control excessive hair growth in women Used in facial steam to help cleanse and tighten pores
Squalane	Increases spreadability of lotions Colorless, transparent and fragrance free
Stearalkonium Chloride	Ammonium compound Adds shine to hair Improves ability to comb hair Conditioning ingredient that forms a

protective coating on the cuticle
Retards tangling
Assist with manageability

Stearic Acid

From animal fats – white, waxy powder
Melted to clear liquid it provides a thick, stiff texture to creams and aids in keeping oils and waters together
Emulsifier (primary purpose – most common use)
Known for the pearly or waxy feel it adds to creams
Ultimately has a cooling effect when applied to skin

Strawberry

Has a natural PH like skin
Mild, effective treatment for all skin types
Nourishing as a soap or lotion component

Strawberry Leaves

Bleaching action
High in Vitamin C
Acidic astringent
Mild anti septic

Sunflower Oil

Moisturizes and regenerates surface cells
Vitamin A & E rich
Protects skin from ultraviolet light
Prevents cell damage from free radicals
Wrinkle fighting

Tamanu nut

Healing to serious skin problems
Used on scrapes, cuts, burns, insect bites and stings, acne, acne scars, psoriasis, diabetic sores, anal fissures, sunburn, dry or scaly skin, blisters, eczema, diaper rash, herpes sores
Treats dry, irritated, mature skin
Promotes healthy, clear, blemish-free skin
Helps clear acne

Fades acne scars
Antimicrobial, antibacterial and anti-fungal
Effective on scabies, ringworm, and athletes foot, jock itch

Tincture

Herbal preparations make with alcohol
Gives longer shelf life to product

Tincture of Benzoin

From gum resin
Used as a preservative
Emulsifier
Some antiseptic properties

Titanium Dioxide

Cream that blocks the suns rays
Use micro-encapsulated kind for easier mixing
White, odorless powder pigment of crystalline structure
High refractive index
Water resistant
Provides long-term UV-protection
Insoluble but dispersible in water and oils

Triethanlamine (TEA)

Emulsifier that works with stearic acid

Vinegar

Derived from fermented fruit juices
Aids in removing reside from the hair
Acts as a clarifying agent when mixed with water
Vinegar is a STRONG substance that can be damaging when applied directly
MUST BE DILUTED

Vitamin A

Beta Carotene
Causes orange color in cosmetics
Vitamin A
Antioxidant - aids removing free radicals
Encourages collagen production - causes

the skin to plump out
*** Monitor use carefully as too much can cause damage

Vitamin B

Cumulative conditioning effects in hair products with extended, regular use
Absorbed by the hair to protect form atmospheric conditions

Vitamin C

Found in many fruits and vegetables
Acts as a preservative and anti-oxidant

Vitamin E

Natural preservative
Emollient
AMA – make skin softer, smoother, reduces roughness, cracking and irritation
May retard signs of aging

Vodka

Derived from potato and grains
Used in cosmetics for hair
Acts as a solvent
Product Base

Watercress

Juice has a mild acid that contains iron, minerals and phosphorus
Clarifying agent for oily hair – removes soap residue and oils

Water Dock Root

Used in ointment or shampoo to treat scalp conditions – dandruff

Watermelon Oil

Dissolves Sebum

WAXES

Beeswax

Derived from the secretions of bees when they are forming honeycombs
Forms a protective barrier on the hair
Provides a guard against environmental

factors
Anti-bacterial
Tames fly-away hair
Used in straightening agents
Repels moisture – limits frizz or curl
Cuticles – provides protection, sooths
frayed torn cuticles
Emulsifier and stiffener

Candelilla Wax

From candelilla plant, a desert shrub
native to New Mexico and Texas
Thickener (can be used to replace
beeswax)

Carnauba Wax

From leaves of Brazilian wax palm tree
Melting point is 181 degrees
Extremely hard wax for hard set recipes
Emulsifying Wax

Polawax

Plant based
Emulsifier – used to create bond between
water and oil
Good in lotions and creams
Makes a fluid cream and lotion without
separation
Nice end texture

Jasmine Wax

Floral wax from jasmine distillation
Fragrant thickener

Wheat Germ Oil

High in Vitamin A, B1, D, lecithin, protein
and fatty acids
Very high Vitamin E
Very emollient – needs mixed to remove
sticky
Preservative

Wheat Protein

Hydrolyzed (turned partly into water) =
nitrogen carrying

Beneficial to hair = protein
Add gloss, body and luster to hair
Deposits a protective film on the that is
smoothing and moisturizing

Witch Hazel   Astringent that can be used on irritated
skin
Calms itchy uncomfortable skin

Xanthan Gum   Natural sugar
Gel Thickener
Thickens and stabilizes products but
difficult to work with because it does not
dissolve in water

Yarrow Root   Contains azulens
Anti-inflammatory
Reduces effect of unbroken blemishes

Yogurt   Made from fermented milk combined
with bacteria
Skin softener

Zinc Oxide   *** Purchase only USP grade intended for
cosmetic use
Antibacterial, antiseptic, astringent
Protective
Can be used as a sun screen
Encourages healing
White pigment

Appendix B Recipe Locator

www.ingramcontent.com/pod-product-compliance
Lightning Source LLC
Chambersburg PA
CBHW081824280526

45789CB00007B/2332